*This book will revolutionize the treatment of learning disorders. Learn all about*

- A major breakthrough in treating the three leading learning disorders—how it happened, what it means, how you can use it now
- LCP—long chain polyunsaturated fatty acid supplementation: what it is, why it's healthy, how it dramatically improves the lives of handicapped children and adults
- Increasing your child's intake of LCPs through simple supplementation and dietary changes
- ADHD—recognizing the warning signs, and the astonishing steps you can take to help your child's concentration and behavior
- Dyslexia—the myths and facts: heredity factors, correlation with intelligence, taking effective action at home and at school
- Dyspraxia—why it is often unrecognized, and simple strategies for helping cope with this "clumsy child syndrome"
- Guidance, advice, resources, and real-life stories that address all your concerns

# THE LCP SOLUTION

## The Remarkable Nutritional Treatment for ADHD, Dyslexia, and Dyspraxia

**B. JACQUELINE STORDY, Ph.D.,**
**and MALCOLM J. NICHOLL**

BALLANTINE BOOKS · NEW YORK

# CONTENTS

# INTRODUCTION

My son is dyslexic. With the benefit of hindsight I'm sure that my father, an exceptionally bright and talented man, was also dyslexic. Other close family members have various learning disorders, and I believe I have a mild form of dyslexia myself. I hate to write, that's for sure.

Learning disorders *do* run in families, and mine is no exception. It's true, too, that many, many people with learning challenges are amazingly talented, creative, and entrepreneurial. They are people who have achieved the pinnacles of success in their chosen careers—whether politicians, scientists, businessmen, and, yes, even writers—in spite of having what might be considered an overwhelming handicap.

My personal experience has given me a valuable insight into the lives of those individuals who face the day-to-day ordeal of living with attention deficit/hyperactivity disorder (ADHD), dyslexia, and dyspraxia. It has also instilled in me a genuine empathy and immense regard for all of those children whose lives are touched by a problem that has them offhandedly dismissed as unruly, dumb, lazy, or clumsy.

It's especially distressing when the reality is that such youngsters begin life with the deck stacked against them, that they have a biological predisposition to their personal learning disorder. These youngsters have a genetic imprint making it so much harder for them to pay attention, to learn to read and write, to be coordinated, or to excel on the sports field.

There was a point when my personal and professional experiences interfaced, one of those "lightbulb" events—a crystallizing moment. It began when my son, James, at the age of seven, was identified as having dyslexia. He was obviously intelligent, but he was not performing in school to the level everyone expected. He had a phenomenal vocabulary, but his reading was not up to his age group and his spelling, quite frankly, could only be described as bizarre.

When he was diagnosed as dyslexic it made me think of my own challenges. Even today, I can vividly remember being asked, in primary school, to write a paragraph and panicking with every word I struggled to put on the page. As I got older, I managed to learn the rules of spelling, punctuation, and grammar that seem to dyslexic children like the code of some secret society to which they have not been admitted. Verbally, I have never had any difficulty whatsoever. I spent more than thirty wonderful years teaching dietitians and nutritionists at the largest undergraduate program of its kind in Europe. I thoroughly enjoyed putting thoughts together into a constructive argument, as well as explaining sophisticated and complex scientific research. I still do. But I've always disliked writing, and that continues to be a real burden.

My aversion to writing reminds me of my father. He left school at an early age during the Great Depression. Later, in his twenties, he talked his way into a university engineering course, even though he didn't have the appropriate qualifications. As I've subsequently discovered, that's a typical dyslexic approach—

verbal and convincing. My father was very entrepreneurial, and went on to successfully build his own business, notwithstanding his poor skills with the written word.

And then came James. When he was diagnosed as dyslexic, it prompted me to reflect not only about my father and myself, but also about my whole family history. Other close relatives are extremely intelligent, but nevertheless have signs of learning disorders that were never officially recognized. One day it occurred to me that relatives who had been breast-fed the longest were less affected by dyslexia than those who had not been breast-fed at all, or had been breast-fed for a relatively short period.

What was the connection?

Mother's milk, of course, is the ultimate nourishment for a newborn baby, containing specific fatty acids critical, in particular, for brain and visual development. The brain itself is comprised of 60 percent fat and major components are the long-chain polyunsaturated fatty acids (LCPs) that are the primary focus of this book. These LCPs are, in effect, the building blocks of the all-important phospholipid membranes around and within nerve cells. Every human thought and every human action that originates inside the awesomely elaborate human brain can only occur when the brain receives the nutritional support of the LCPs. One of these LCPs, docosahexaenoic acid (DHA), is also a major constituent of membranes in the cone and rod cells of the retina and is, therefore, vital for eyesight.

For a person to read and write effectively requires sensory input from vision, hearing, or touch, and central processing in the brain. The ability to write requires messages from the brain being relayed by motor nerves to the muscles of the hand. So, taking all of this into account, I began to wonder if some kind of disorder of fatty acid metabolism could be implicated in dyslexia. This was the trigger that initiated my investigation into the potential role of LCPs in learning disorders. My initial research with dyslexics led to further study with dyspraxic children (or as the condition is officially titled, developmental coordination disorder). At the same time, in the United States, pivotal research along the same lines, but with ADHD children, was under way at Purdue University, spearheaded by John Burgess and Laura Stevens.

Intriguingly, a common genetic basis to ADHD, dyslexia, and dyspraxia is strongly indicated as all of these conditions tend to run in the same families and are often co-morbid—that is, they occur together. That common basis, in the studies conducted so far, strongly suggests a defect in fatty acid metabolism, and that these learning disorders can be improved when an individual is supplemented with LCPs. Studies at Oxford University, using brain scans to peer inside the active brains of dyslexic patients, have now provided support for this proposition.

In the wider world of research, other clues have emerged. There is now plentiful evidence of a deficiency of LCPs in the modern diet. This is the direct result of a change in our eating habits (through manufacturing processes and by choice), and a reduction in the numbers of mothers breast-feeding. Within the same time frame—the last one hundred years—corresponding to the decrease in LCP intake there has been a dramatic *increase* in learning disorders. Further studies—including double-blind, placebo-controlled trials—are already in progress, but I am confident that a doorway has been opened that can lead to a meaningful difference in the lives of the tens of millions of people afflicted with ADHD, dyslexia, and dyspraxia.

In this book I provide the scientific evidence gathered to date—much of it in just the last couple of years. I also share with you the experiences of health professionals in the field, and some of the touching stories of children whose lives have already been transformed as a result of LCP supplementation. In my view, there is compelling data indicating that a new solution to the problems experienced by many sufferers of ADHD, dyslexia, and dyspraxia is now at hand. But that is not all. In addition, I provide other nutritional and educational information to help people with learning disorders and the families who support them.

—B. JACQUELINE STORDY, PH.D.

As far as I was concerned, kids with attention deficit/hyperactivity disorder were the troublemakers who couldn't sit still and who turned classrooms into chaos. Dyslexics were just children who couldn't read very well, couldn't construct sentences, wrote their letters backwards. Dyspraxia? Developmental coordination disorder? Like 95 percent of the population, I'd never heard of this condition, although I was familiar with extremely clumsy children who were the proverbial accidents waiting to happen.

Then, Dr. Jacqueline Stordy, a scientist I'd known and respected for more than a decade, told me about her fascinating research and that of other experts in the field. I was immediately hooked. As a professional writer since my teens, I was intrigued by the thought of investigating the painful predicament of individuals who found it hard to read the simple sentences of a tabloid newspaper, or to construct a brief, legible letter.

So much of society today is based on the ability to acquire and use information, to read books, surf the Internet, write reports, correspond quickly and efficiently not just office to office but country to country—and all at the press of a button. What was it like to be disenfranchised from this world? What was it like to be isolated from communicating effectively with one's peers? Interesting questions. Interesting subject. From a purely objective standpoint I was curious and anxious to learn more. Unlike Dr. Stordy, I had had no direct personal experience of any of these learning disorders. But what started as an academic and journalistic exercise became much more. When you hear the heart-wrenching stories of parents struggling to come to terms with their children's learning handicaps, you cannot help but experience an emotional charge. You ask yourself, "How on earth do they cope? How do they manage?"

By and large, the unsung heroes are the parents, who see beyond their own child's learning disorder and rise to the challenge. Parents who dedicate themselves to searching out the best approach for their child, who know that beyond the frustrating inability of the moment is a child with long-term, lifelong potential. The determination and resilience of these parents impressed and awed me. But when I fully investigated the work of Dr. Stordy and so many other professional researchers—at highly respected universities and hospitals—new emotions came into force. For now there is hope. Hope that children with ADHD, dyslexia, and dyspraxia can have their conditions vastly improved.

To my knowledge, this is the first book that has identified and tackled the overlap and interconnection between ADHD, dyslexia, and the lesser-known disorder of dyspraxia, which is much more prevalent than you might imagine. It really took the discovery of a nutritional solution to these distressing problems to highlight the commonalties. Dr. Stordy is the first to say that we are at the beginning, and that all of the answers are by no means available. Finding the ultimate solution is, as she so expressively puts it, like constructing "a three-dimensional jigsaw." But now there are significant indicators that the kind of supplementation with LCPs advocated by Dr. Stordy and her colleagues is more than merely promising. It's exciting, and it's a phenomenal advance that gives great new hope to everyone who is "learning challenged."

—MALCOLM J. NICHOLL

# CHAPTER 1

# ALL IN THE FAMILY

*The fact that learning disabilities tend to run in families indicates that there may be a genetic link.*
—FROM THE NATIONAL INSTITUTE OF MENTAL HEALTH BOOKLET *LEARNING DISABILITIES*

They are the hidden handicaps. There are no crutches, no wheelchairs, no braces, and no physical characteristics that distinguish them in a crowd. There is no sign at all that behind the seemingly ordinary facade lies a serious debilitating impediment. Children (and adults) with ADHD, dyslexia, and dyspraxia look just like regular folk. It's easy, therefore, to dismiss them as "space cadets," "whirling dervishes," "motor mouths," "dingdongs," "hostile," "lazy," "dumb," "clumsy," or whatever convenient slur readily springs to mind. It's all too easy to criticize, to squarely lay the onus on such individuals as if they have deliberately, even provocatively, made a conscious decision to behave this way, when the truth is that they don't have a choice in the matter.

Yet until very recently some health and education professionals have disputed the very existence of such learning disorders.

1

Even today, there is still some disagreement over the exact criteria by which we should recognize these problems. But there is ever-growing scientific proof validating the very real existence of this trio of troubles. There is substantial evidence, too, of their serious impact on individual families and society as a whole.

As the twentieth century came to a close, it was apparent that learning disorders are widespread in the Western world. In the United States, the National Institutes of Health (NIH) estimates that as much as 15 to 20 percent of the population suffers from one or more of the principal learning disorders. ADHD, for instance, has even been called an "epidemic" and the "fastest growing childhood disorder in the United States." In fact, in the United States, a threefold increase in the prevalence of learning disorders was noted between 1976 and 1993. Some 17.5 million American children cope with learning problems of one kind or another.

The effect this has on their lives can be profound. According to the National Center for Learning Disabilities, a nonprofit organization:

- Adolescents with learning disabilities are at great risk of abusing drugs and alcohol. In one study, as many as 60 percent of youngsters receiving treatment for substance abuse suffered from a learning handicap.
- Thirty-five percent of students afflicted with a learning disability do not finish high school. (The number is actually much higher because many others drop out without their learning disadvantage having been officially identified.)
- Some 62 percent of students with learning disabilities do not have a full-time job one year after graduating from high school.

Vulnerable to drug and alcohol abuse. Likely to drop out of high school. Just as likely to be out of work. These are only some of the misfortunes that individuals with learning challenges have to shoulder. ADHD children, in particular, grow up to have more health problems, more encounters with the law, more traffic accidents, and more risky sexual escapades.

The problem is getting worse. An increasing number of children and adults are being diagnosed with these ailments. Why? The greater incidence, of course, may simply reflect greater awareness and better diagnosis, but, as you'll discover, changes in food manufacturing processes and dietary habits, as well as a decline in breast-feeding, have all played a major role. These changes, which began in the early 1900s, have accelerated at an alarming pace within the last twenty years.

## A FAMILY AFFAIR

It's in the genes! Your family history largely predetermines your chances of inheriting a learning disorder, just as much as it indicates a predisposition to cancer, diabetes, and other physical diseases. It has long been recognized that learning disorders such as ADHD, dyslexia, and dyspraxia run in families. In fact, it is not at all unusual to find a family that has one child with ADHD, another with dyslexia, and a third with dyspraxia. It is also quite common for individuals to suffer from more than one of these conditions.

In fact:

- As many as 65 percent of children with ADHD also struggle with at least one other learning disorder, and sometimes bipolar disorder and/or Tourette's syndrome.
- Fifty percent of dyspraxic children also have ADHD, according to one study of more than four hundred seven-year-olds.
- Some 30 to 50 percent of children with dyslexia have

ADHD, and vice versa. The Dyslexia Research Institute puts the number even higher, saying that 60 percent of ADHD children also have dyslexia.

But what exactly are these learning disorders that challenge our children from their earliest formative years and haunt many of them for the rest of their lives? They are all, in fact, complex neurological conditions that occur, by and large, in children of at least average intelligence; many are actually above average. Simplistically put, their brains are "wired" somewhat differently. It is also well known that when you have conditions such as ADHD, dyslexia, and dyspraxia, which co-exist, it's very likely that underlying them all is a common genetic and biological basis.

## ADHD

ADHD is characterized by persistent and excessive problems in which the child is unable to focus and pay attention, or conversely displays hyperactive and impulsive behavior. Many children manage to combine both aspects. An association with dyslexia seems to be stronger for children with the inattentive rather than the hyperactive type of ADHD.

## Dyslexia

Dyslexia is an inherent dysfunction involving the language centers of the brain. Children who have had appropriate schooling and appear intelligent encounter an unexpected difficulty in reading, spelling, and writing. The spoken word may be affected to some degree, but the handicap is particularly related to mastering the written word.

## Dyspraxia (and Apraxia)

Also known as developmental coordination disorder, dyspraxia is a disability in which children are slow to achieve many of the normal childhood milestones as the result of an impairment or immaturity in the organization of movement. There may be associated difficulties learning to speak, a condition known as developmental apraxia of speech. Children with this problem find it extremely hard to correctly pronounce sounds, syllables, and words. Some of them are virtually speechless.

---

### ADHD, DYSLEXIA, AND DYSPRAXIA— DEFINING FEATURES

**ADHD**

- Hyperactivity
- Impulsivity
- Attention problems

**Dyslexia**

- Specific problems with written language skills (reading/ spelling/writing)

**Dyspraxia**

- Problems in planning and execution of movements
- Poor motor coordination, attention

---

## MAKING THE CONNECTION

The close relationship between these three disorders has not been properly appreciated. It has been obscured, I suspect, by the differences in the way they have been identified and subsequently treated. Children with ADHD, dyslexia, or dyspraxia are steered into considerably different methods of care in the hands of considerably different kinds of health and education professionals.

Children with ADHD are usually, in the first instance, under the care of a pediatrician. More often than not, the doctor will either prescribe stimulant medication such as Ritalin or he will recommend behavior therapy, or a combination of both. Concerns have been expressed about the massive overprescription of Ritalin in the United States, with allegations that it is being used as a panacea for "bad behavior," and about the long-term effect of such medication, which is unknown. For reasons that will soon become apparent, I support the use of long-chain polyunsaturated fatty acids (LCPs) as the sensible alternative to these drugs. But it is only fair to point out that recent surveys have indicated that the more likely occurrence will be an "underprescription" of Ritalin.

Children with dyslexia usually remain under the wing of the educational psychologist. The inability of these children to master the basic rules for reading and writing has been primarily regarded as a problem to be solved in the classroom. Consequently, attempts to help dyslexic children have focused on educational techniques, including such methods as multisensory learning. Dyspraxic children usually end up in the hands of physical therapists. Their clumsiness and awkwardness have made a combination of physiotherapy and occupational therapy the treatment of choice for them. A regimen of repetitive physical activities has been regarded as the only way to help stimulate and coordinate the movement of their limbs.

## ADHD, DYSLEXIA, AND DYSPRAXIA— COMMON FEATURES

- Neurodevelopmental anomalies
  Pregnancy and birth complications
  Low birth weight, reduced head circumference
  Minor physical anomalies
- Excess of males affected
- Allergies/autoimmune problems
- Other physical complaints, such as stomachache
  and migraine
- Motor coordination problems
- Sleep problems
- Mood disorders
  Depression, mood swings
- Behavioral problems
  Hostility, stress-aggression
  Impulsivity, hyperactivity
- Perceptual and cognitive abnormalities
  Visual and auditory problems
  Attention/working memory

Not surprisingly, with different types of health professionals taking responsibility for these three disorders, scant consideration has been given to any common denominators. Now there's a new school of thought. Diverse scientific undertakings including nutritional studies, extensive genetic research, surveys of close family relatives, and increasingly sophisticated brain imaging techniques have all combined to muster new evidence.

As you'll discover, these specific learning disorders now appear to be associated with an inborn error of metabolism affecting the conversion of shorter-chain essential fatty acids (EFAs) into the longer-chain polyunsaturated fatty acids (LCPs), and the incorporation of sufficient amounts of the latter into cell membranes. This leads to a deficiency of the LCPs required for normal, effective, rapid-fire communication between neurons.

# A CLOSER LOOK AT EACH DISORDER

## ADHD—Twins Provide the Proof

ADHD has been identified in every nation and every culture where it has been investigated. It is estimated that between 2 and 9.5 percent of all school-age children worldwide have ADHD. And it is at least two to three times more prevalent in boys than girls—possibly because boys are genetically more prone to disorders of the nervous system, but also because it is more readily identified in boys. ADHD males are more likely to exhibit hyperactive behavior; ADHD females are more likely to be inattentive. Symptoms of ADHD do continue into adulthood but diminish over the years. Hyperactivity declines more quickly than impulsivity or inattentiveness, says Myron Genel, M.D., professor of pediatrics at Yale University School of Medicine.

Clear evidence that ADHD runs in families comes from studies of twins. In as many as 80 to 90 percent of identical twins (who possess identical genes), if one had ADHD so did the other. In fraternal twins (who have just 25 percent identical genes) the likelihood of both having ADHD drops to 32 to 50 percent. This is many times greater than the incidence among unrelated children. The influence of genes is unmistakable.

A recent large-scale study has supported earlier ADHD research with twins that was carried out at the University of Colorado and the University of Southampton in the United Kingdom. In the April 1999 issue of the *Journal of the American Academy of Child and Adolescent Psychiatry*, researchers at the Washington University School of Medicine in St. Louis, Missouri, reported on their investigation into the incidence of ADHD in more than 2,600 twins. In this study—of children born between 1968 and 1994—identical twins suffered from the same class of ADHD symptoms about 80 percent of the time; fraternal twins matched about 50 percent of the time.

In another study of relatives, researchers at Massachusetts General Hospital looked at 457 parents, brothers, and sisters of 75 children with ADHD. They compared them with the close families of 26 children who had other psychiatric disorders and also the relatives of 26 children with no mental health problems at all. Twenty-five percent of the family members of the ADHD children also had the disorder. Only 5 percent of relatives in the two other groups did.

Furthermore, neurobiological evidence has begun to accumulate confirming the genetic connection signaled by the studies with twins. Scientists have now identified locations on three chromosomes connected with ADHD. Of particular note: Researchers at the University of California at Irvine recently reported finding an abnormal gene associated with ADHD that controls brain receptors of the neurotransmitter dopamine. Children with a more severe form of ADHD have an abnormality of this gene, causing less sensitivity to dopamine. (Ritalin is known to influence dopamine metabolism, which may well account for the drug's efficacy.)

## Dyslexia—A Family History Is Key

Approximately 10 percent of the population in both the United States and the United Kingdom suffer from dyslexia to some extent and 4 percent are severely affected, according to the results of government-sponsored studies. The Dyslexia Research Institute, a national, nonprofit organization, goes further, saying that 10 to 15 percent of the U.S. population has dyslexia, yet only five out of every one hundred dyslexics are recognized and receive attention. The National Institute of Mental Health (NIMH), meanwhile, reports that some 2 to 8 percent of elementary schoolchildren have reading disabilities, most notably dyslexia. An accurate assessment of dyslexia, however, is difficult, as experts cannot even agree on a precise definition of the condition. It used to be believed that dyslexia primarily affected boys, but recent research suggests a more equal balance between the sexes.

Family history is pinpointed as one of the most important risk factors by one of America's leading dyslexia researchers, Sally E. Shaywitz, a professor of pediatrics at Yale University. In a 1998 overview in the *New England Journal of Medicine*, Shaywitz wrote that studies show that from 23 percent to as many as 65 percent of dyslexic children have a parent with the problem, and 40 percent have a brother or sister similarly affected.

Other compelling evidence for a genetic cause comes from a study of twins performed at the University of Colorado in Boulder. In the largest study of its kind, researchers J. C. DeFries and Maricela Alarcon analyzed reading performance data for 186 pairs of identical twins and 138 pairs of same-sex fraternal twins. At least one member of each pair had a reading disability. The researchers' conclusion was that more than half of the reading performance deficit was attributable to heritable influences.

Other research has suggested differences in some regions of the brain between dyslexics and those who are not reading-impaired. Evidence stems from autopsies of the brain as well as sophisticated brain imaging work peering inside the brains of live subjects. Investigators led by Dr. Shaywitz used functional magnetic resonance imaging (fMRI) to produce computer-generated images of the brain while twenty-nine dyslexics and thirty-two nondyslexics performed various reading tasks. They studied seventeen brain regions previously identified as being involved in reading and language and concluded that there were "significant differences in brain activation patterns."

The dyslexic readers showed relative underactivation in regions at the back of the brain (Wernicke's area, the angular gyrus, and striate cortex) and overactivation in a frontal area (inferior frontal gyrus). Says Dr. Shaywitz: "If you have a broken arm, we can see that on an X ray. These brain-activation patterns now provide ... evidence for what has previously been a hidden disability." American University education professor Sally L. Smith expresses it a little more bluntly: "The naysayers used to say there's no such thing as a learning disability, only lazy children. Today, they can see the MRI." Professor Smith adds that MRI technology clearly demonstrates that there is a different architecture in the brains of children with learning disorders. You will see in a later chapter of this book that fMRI has also revealed changes in the chemistry of the brain.

Dr. Shaywitz, who has tracked 451 schoolchildren since 1983 and estimates that some 20 percent of them are reading-disabled, is quick to point out the undoubted accomplishments of many dyslexics in spite of their difficulty in reading. Dyslexia, she says, "has always been a paradox because it may affect reading, but very, very smart and accomplished people can have this problem, including Nobel laureates in science, literature, and other areas."

Apart from studies with twins, by the end of 1999 scientists had identified locations on four separate chromosomes that may be involved in the passing of dyslexia from generation to generation. The latest study pinpointing a new gene for dyslexia located on chromosome 2 appeared in the September 1999 issue of the *Journal of Medical Genetics.* The authors, from the Department of Medical Genetics, University Hospital of Tromsö, Norway, commented: "Since no gene for dyslexia has been isolated, little is known about the molecular processes involved. The isolation and molecular characterization of this newly reported gene on chromosome 2 (DYX3) and DYX1 will thus provide new and exciting insights into the processes involved in reading and spelling." In the rapidly moving world of scientific research, however, their report had barely been published when other researchers came out with a paper proposing mechanisms for the molecular processes involved. The suggestion now is that there is an association with genes that have been linked with altered fat metabolizing enzymes in both dyslexia and ADHD (see table on page 16).

## Dyspraxia—Out of the Shadows

Lesser known than ADHD and dyslexia, dyspraxia affects as many as 6 percent of children between the ages of five and eleven, and deserves far greater attention than it has received. Officially described in the American Psychiatric Association's *DSM-IV* manual as a developmental coordination disorder, dyspraxia's essential feature is a marked impairment in the development of motor coordination (movement skills).

For a diagnosis to be made, the impairment must significantly interfere with academic achievement or normal everyday activities, and the child's abilities must be below what would be expected for his age. The diagnosis is not made if the coordination difficulties are due to a general medical condition such as cerebral palsy or muscular dystrophy.

The manifestations of the disorder vary with age and development and are quite often dismissed in the earlier years on the basis that the child is "just a little bit behind." Younger children may display clumsiness and delays in achieving developmental motor milestones such as walking, crawling, sitting, tying shoelaces, buttoning shirts, and zipping pants. Older children may drop things, be generally clumsy, and have difficulty assembling puzzles, building models, and playing ball. They will also be awkward at printing or handwriting. The disorder is usually first recognized when the child attempts such tasks as running, holding a knife and fork, buttoning clothes, or playing ball games. In some cases, it continues through adolescence and adulthood, though as the individual gets older he is able to make various accommodations in lifestyle so that the problem is not always so evident.

What about a genetic connection? It is highly likely that genes play just as much a part in the occurrence of dyspraxia as they do in ADHD and dyslexia. No research has as yet identified any of the genes, although this is probably as much a reflection of the general dearth of research into dyspraxia as anything else.

## Apraxia—More Than Tongue-tied

Developmental apraxia of speech is also a neurologically based disorder, but exactly how the brain is impaired and what causes the disorder are still unknown. In most instances, there are no obvious clues in a child's prenatal or birth histories. In apraxic children, the area of the brain that instructs the muscles to do what's necessary to make sounds and words come forth is malfunctioning. Therefore, receiving and implementing the "motor plan" for talking runs into a roadblock, in the same way that dyspraxic children don't get the motor plan for bodily coordination.

Generally, in an apraxic child's face, there is nothing wrong with the muscles that need to be manipulated for speech—the tongue, lips, and jaw—and usually the child has no difficulty with nonspeech activities such as chewing and swallowing. (Some apraxic children, however, do have such difficulty, which is particularly unfortunate as it makes it hard for them to swallow beneficial LCP supplements.)

Frustratingly for the apraxic child, she often has a good understanding of language, even though she cannot verbally express herself. She will know what she wants to say, but just cannot make the words come out. If she is able to make a sound at all, it is likely to be the wrong one. Quite often, the child will produce a word or a sound one day, and then not be able to do it the following day. She will also use a simple, single syllable to represent many different words.

When she improves and begins to talk, her language will tend to become inconsistent. She may master individual words, but when putting them together into a short sentence may drop all of the ending sounds. Apraxic children can usually repeat words back to you when prompted much more easily than spontaneously finding them for themselves. The frustration of not being able to speak can make apraxic children aggressive. They may choose to communicate with punches and shoves instead of the words that they are unable to form. In sharp contrast, older children may turn inward and become shy or escape conversations with a standard "I don't know" response.

A child with developmental apraxia of speech needs help. This is not a problem that she will outgrow by herself. Intensive speech therapy is necessary as soon as the disorder is identified, and will need to continue for years. Her communication skills may improve as she gets older, but her speech will continue to be riddled with mistakes, and she will still be difficult to understand.

In this book, I am principally focusing on ADHD, dyslexia, and dyspraxia because actual clinical trials with LCP supplementation have been conducted with regard to these learning disorders. However, there are so many inspiring accounts of apraxic youngsters being successfully supplemented that you will also meet some of them in the pages to come.

What about the genetic factor? So far only one location on one chromosome has been connected with the development of apraxia of speech. It's a start. It's more than has been achieved with dyspraxia, but not yet equivalent to the research into ADHD and dyslexia.

## WHAT ABOUT THOSE GENES?

At this stage, I would like to briefly explore the subject of genetic research. It's complicated, but it is of such fundamental significance that it really helps to forge an understanding of genes and how they affect the way our bodies work. Every cell in the human body contains forty-six chromosomes. These are very long strands of a chemical called DNA (deoxyribonucleic acid), together with protein and some other substances. Half of the chromosome material comes from your father and half from your mother. Genes are regions on the chromosomes, and we have about fifty thousand of them.

Genes send coded messages to other parts of the cell to make specific proteins. The proteins may be those that make up the structure of tissues, such as muscle, or they may be proteins such as enzymes that regulate the chemical reactions needed for growth, energy release, and repair of tissues. There is a huge research effort under way called the human genome project in which scientists worldwide are mapping all of the genes and investigating what chemical processes each controls. The positions on chromosomes that are linked with particular enzymes are identified by certain letters and numbers. These are a bit like identifying where a house is located on a street.

Preliminary research has identified the chromosomes and some of the locations of the genes for ADHD, dyslexia, and verbal dyspraxia (apraxia). Dr. David Horrobin, one of the world experts in essential fatty acid (EFA) metabolism, and his colleague Crispin Bennett have reviewed the scientific literature and linked some of the locations with specific enzymes. The enzymes are variously involved in fatty acid and membrane metabolism.

| | Chromosome | Gene Location | Enzyme |
|---|---|---|---|
| Dyslexia | 1 | p36-p34 | Phospholipase A2 |
| | 2 | p15-p16 | |
| | 6 | p23-p21.3 | Fatty acid–CoA transferase |
| | 15 | q21 | Fatty acid–CoA ligase |
| ADHD | 6 | p21.3 | Fatty acid–CoA transferase |
| | 16 | q11.1-q13 | Phospholipase C |
| | 20 | p11-p12 | Phospholipase C |
| Verbal dyspraxia | 7 | q31 | |

What does all this mean? Enzymes that are called transferase and ligase (as listed in the table) are associated with the incorporation of fatty acids into membranes, whereas the phospholipases are associated with the breakdown of phospholipid membranes. Phospholipids are the building blocks of brain cell membranes, so it is very important that both of these processes are in balance.

It is not just the genes that control how our body chemistry works; sometimes environmental factors interact with our genetic predisposition. Nutrition is one such environmental factor, and it has a strong bearing on how our genes influence our bodies.

In Chapter 5 I will explain how the shorter chain EFAs are converted to the long-chain polyunsaturated fatty acids (LCPs), the important fatty acids that are the building blocks of nerve cell membranes. You can get LCPs direct from a few foods (mainly fish) or your body can make them from EFAs (found in vegetable oils). The efficiency of your body's ability to make LCPs from EFAs is determined by your genes. If you have a genetic problem that makes it difficult for you to convert EFAs into LCPs, you will suffer from an LCP deficiency unless your diet is rich in the foods containing the preformed LCPs.

Let me share with you an anecdotal experience in support of this proposition. When I was lecturing in Montreal, Canada, I was explaining how the Inuit, in general, appear to have difficulty in converting EFAs to LCPs and, therefore, must eat foods rich in LCPs to remain healthy. I was also explaining how dyslexia might be linked to a deficiency of the LCPs. At the end of my lecture a woman in the audience said I had explained something that had happened in her family. She was an Inuit and had a dyslexic daughter. The daughter had not been breast-fed and, as a result, had not received LCPs as a baby. As a child and young adult she had not eaten much fish, so throughout these critical years of growth and development her diet had been deficient in LCPs. As a young adult, she had returned to her ethnic origins and had eaten the traditional Inuit diet of fish that naturally contains significant amounts of the LCPs. Subsequently, her dyslexic symptoms improved dramatically. But when she returned to Montreal, and once again consumed a typical North American diet, her dyslexic condition worsened again.

## IN SUMMARY

Three common learning disorders, one common bond. There is no doubt that ADHD, dyslexia, and dyspraxia run in families. There is no doubt that some children are afflicted with two—

sometimes even all three—of these handicaps. It is time that health and education professionals recognized the interrelationship so that the most effective treatments can be introduced in the earliest years of these children's lives.

Behavior therapy, multisensory teaching techniques, physiotherapy, and occupational therapy are all important strategies. But genetic research has indicated that a problem of fat metabolism may be involved. So, what about nutrition? What about the most fundamental "treatment" of all—ensuring that children are fed "brain-healthy" foods? What about ensuring that those children who have "faulty wiring" are supplemented with the right kind of nutrition to ensure that the brain's messaging system functions properly?

In the following pages you'll be introduced to the mushrooming research in the United States, Europe, and elsewhere pointing to the need for the brain to be nourished with long-chain polyunsaturated fatty acids (LCPs). You'll also meet some of the children whose lives have already been transformed through nutritional supplementation. But first we need to review exactly what we are dealing with and take a look at the state of knowledge that exists with regard to the history of ADHD, dyslexia, and dyspraxia. Furthermore, it is important to look at the real impact these disorders have on the lives of children and their families, and what has been done so far to treat them.

# THE DISORDERS

# CHAPTER 2

# ADHD—What We Know So Far

*Children with attention deficit disorders are like diamonds in the rough: It takes special care and time for them to dazzle.*
—Nancy S. Boyles and Darlene Contadino, *Parenting a Child with Attention Deficit/Hyperactivity Disorder*

It is a typical morning in the Thompson household. Seven-year-old Mike, an angelic picture of innocence when he is asleep, awakes at 6:00—and hurls himself into the day. When his mother calls him for breakfast, Mike stomps into the kitchen, grabs a box of cornflakes, and liberally spills the cereal all over the table. Then he crunches the cornflakes into little pieces, all the while relentlessly kicking the table leg. He can't sit still. He dashes outside, collects the morning newspaper from the front step, and before his father can intervene, Mike has managed to shred the news of the day.

Mike's mother—with a calm authority born out of long-suffering experience—orders him to get a dustpan and brush and clean up the mess. Mike dutifully heads to the closet and gets the utensils, but then he can't remember what he's supposed to do with them. Instead, he buries himself in a box containing an assortment of cleaning materials, and loses himself in a world of his own. When his mother reminds him of his assigned task, he storms back to his room, slamming doors behind him, and spends the next fifteen minutes playing soccer with anything he can kick. Young Mike has an extreme form of attention deficit/hyperactivity disorder (ADHD) that hasn't been treated.

Mike's behavior doesn't improve once he gets to school. He's restless, constantly on the move, squirming in his seat. He annoys his teachers and classmates by blurting out answers to questions, even before the questions have been completed. He interrupts conversations and talks incessantly. Instead of concentrating on the blackboard, he's looking out the window at a blackbird and conjuring up an incredible fantasy. Mike's not mentally present in the classroom. As far as he's concerned, he's flying with the blackbird on an adventure searching for hidden treasure in some mystical kingdom far beyond the mountains.

That's typical, says Barbara D. Ingersoll, Ph.D., author of *Distant Drums, Different Drummers. A Guide for Young People with ADHD:* "When people with ADHD have to pay attention to things they find dull, they often create their own excitement. They may dream about action heroes and come up with new ideas for an exciting plot, scary monsters or powerful weapons. Sometimes, in fact, they become so interested in developing new adventures or sketching new weapons that an entire lesson goes by and they don't hear a word the teacher says."

When it's time to play games, Mike won't wait until it's his turn and barges ahead of the other children. For him, absorbing and following instructions is impossible, He's always losing things—books, pencils, clothes. Perhaps worst of all, he frequently engages in dangerous and reckless activities such as climbing trees, rushing into traffic, and jumping from high places (more than the average child does)—all without considering the consequences to himself or others. He throws caution to the wind, acting first and thinking later—when it is probably too late and someone has been physically or emotionally hurt, or something has been destroyed.

Mike pushes and shoves people out of the way because he is so single-minded in his pursuit of something that he wants. He has great difficulty following rules. He's a "repeat offender" who doesn't learn from experience. He's a chronic underachiever. He is actually very intelligent, but it's sheer torture for him to sit still and pay attention to an exam paper, so his grades are not a true reflection of his ability. (Mike's not alone. By adolescence, as many as one-third of children with ADHD will have failed at least one grade in school.)

Mike displays both the hyperactive-impulsive *and* inattentive forms of ADHD. There are children with some—even all—of these same character traits, although maybe not quite so outlandish as in Mike's case. Imagine, however, when there is more than one ADHD child in a home or a classroom. A couple of children in a class who have undiagnosed or untreated ADHD can create bedlam, and turn a thoughtful, enthusiastic, caring teacher into a burned-out wreck. They're the kids no one wants to invite to a birthday party; they're the kids baby-sitters dread.

Parents of ADHD children with the predominantly hyperactive condition certainly have to be hyperalert. Children like Mike are more likely to impulsively engage in risky activities, and act on challenges from their friends, perhaps from a need to be accepted. They have a hard time keeping still, especially in places where it is most often required, such as in the classroom, church, or a restaurant. Children with ADHD are frequently implored to "try harder." They're urged, "If you would only work harder you'd do better." But this kind of pressure often backfires. The harder they try, the more disorganized they get, and the more frustrated they become, until they reach the point where they flatly give up.

The social consequences of having ADHD are often neglected. There's more to the disability than getting poor grades in school or performing inadequately at work. To make friends you need to be able to conform to social etiquette. You need to be able to follow what is being said in a group discussion, to be able to pay attention. Subtle social cues, especially body language, can be totally missed by the person with ADHD: the raising of eyebrows, narrowing of eyes, pursing of lips, slight change in voice tone, tilting of the head. Being oblivious to these signals can lead to social gaffes or a sense of isolation.

## GIRLS GET IT, TOO

How prevalent is ADHD? It is conservatively estimated that 3 to 5 percent of the childhood population in the United States has ADHD, and as much as half continue to be affected into adulthood. In total, at least 17 million people in the United States have ADHD. Typically thought of as a condition that strikes boys—it is two to three times more common in boys—ADHD also affects young girls. Girls are generally less readily identified because they tend to demonstrate more of the inattention symptoms, which are less obvious than boys' hyperactivity. According to a 1999 study funded by the National Institute of Mental Health (NIMH)—the largest and most comprehensive study of girls so far—the correlates between girls and boys were remarkably similar. Among the few differences: The girls were less likely to have a co-existing behavior disorder, but they were two and a half times more likely to have problems related to substance abuse. A study in the June 2000 issue of the journal *Pediatrics* found an increase in the diagnosis of ADHD from 1.4 per cent to 9.2 percent between 1979 and

1996. This was based on a survey of more than 21,000 patients aged between four and fifteen, reported by Dr. Kelly Kelleher and colleagues at the University of Pittsburgh.

ADHD is a multifaceted condition. Everyone with ADHD does not behave in the same way. Some are quiet dreamers who disappear into their own worlds and display no signs of hyperactivity. Others are human dynamos, bouncing off the walls, a frenzy of activity. Still others are impatient, constantly interrupt conversations, and are always on the lookout for new stimulating activities. Often, they are described as "novelty junkies."

"Imagine living in a fast-moving kaleidoscope, where sounds, images and thoughts are constantly shifting, feeling easily bored, yet helpless to keep your mind on tasks you need to complete," says an ADHD booklet published by the NIMH. "Distracted by unimportant sights and sounds, your mind drives you from one thought or activity to the next. Perhaps you are so wrapped up in a collage of thoughts and images that you don't notice when someone speaks to you."

ADHD sufferers who have the predominantly inattentive condition talk about getting sidetracked all the time, never being able to finish tasks, drifting off onto some other activity, completely forgetting what they had originally begun to do. They're consistently inconsistent. Psychologist and author Paul L. Weingartner provides the analogy of a television remote control whose batteries are low: "Sometimes they work normally, and sometimes you have to push the button over and over again before the battery sends enough current to change the channel. . . . A friend may call you and urge you to turn to a certain channel because something important is on. You push the buttons but nothing happens. As the person on the phone rushes you to change the channel, you shake the remote control, push some other buttons desperately, and, just then, the battery delivers enough power to change to another channel that you do not really want."

We've all experienced frustrations like that from time to time. For the person with ADHD, however, it is a daily occurrence, something he lives with all the time. Asked a question by his teacher, the ADHD child may not remember one or more critical elements. His anxiety rises as he frantically gropes for the right answer. Rather than not answer at all, he take a wild stab at it and is way off target. He's on a different wavelength. The rest of the class dissolves in laughter.

## In the Beginning

ADHD was first defined by British pediatrician George Frederic Still in a series of lectures to the Royal College of Physicians in 1902, and later published in the prestigious British medical journal *The Lancet*. In the verbose language of his time, Still described a group of twenty young patients who showed signs of "lawlessness," lacked "inhibitory volition," and were generally "obstreperous, dishonest and willful." Even then, Still hypothesized that the condition was not the result of bad parenting or "moral turpitude" but was either biologically inherited or due to injury at birth.

Over the years, a variety of labels have been attached to children with the condition, including such terms as "minimal brain dysfunction," "brain-injured child syndrome," "hyperkinetic reaction of childhood," and "hyperactive child syndrome"—reflecting successive generations of physicians' uncertainty about the exact cause of the disorder. The term "attention deficit disorder" became widely used in the 1980s. Today, the official name is attention deficit/hyperactivity disorder (ADHD).

The American Psychiatric Association's reference book, the *Diagnostic and Statistical Manual of Mental Disorders*, fourth edition (*DSM-IV*), is responsible for the latest labeling. The main categories of ADHD are:

- predominantly inattentive
- predominantly hyperactive-impulsive
- a combination of the two

What are the criteria for diagnosing ADHD? The manual tells specialists to assess whether the behavior is persistent, as well as excessive and more prevalent, compared to others of the same age. The behavior also needs to occur in varied settings (both at home and at school, for example) and some of the symptoms need to have appeared before the age of seven.

According to the *DSM*, a diagnosis of ADHD/inattentive type can be made if six or more of the following symptoms have often been displayed for at least six months:

1. failing to pay close attention to details or making careless mistakes in schoolwork or other activities
2. difficulty sustaining attention in tasks or play activities
3. not seeming to listen when spoken to directly
4. not following through on instructions and failing to finish schoolwork or chores
5. difficulty organizing tasks or activities
6. avoids, dislikes, or is reluctant to engage in tasks that require sustained mental effort (such as schoolwork or homework)
7. loses things such as toys, school assignments, pencils, books, and tools
8. easily distracted by extraneous stimuli
9. forgetful in daily activities

A diagnosis of ADHD/hyperactivity-impulsivity can be made if six or more of the following symptoms have often been displayed for at least six months:

### Hyperactivity

1. fidgets with hands or feet or squirms in seat
2. leaves seat in classroom or other settings in which re-maining seated is expected
3. runs about or climbs excessively in inappropriate situations
4. difficulty playing or engaging in leisure activities quietly
5. "on the go" or acts as if "driven by a motor"
6. talks excessively

### Impulsivity

7. blurts out answers before questions have been completed
8. has difficulty awaiting turn
9. interrupts or intrudes on others by, for example, butting into conversations or games

Remember, the above behaviors must occur frequently and in more than one setting.

A diagnosis of ADHD/combined type can be made if six (or more) symptoms of inattention and six (or more) symptoms of hyperactivity impulsivity have persisted for at least six months. Interestingly, *most* children and adolescents with ADHD have the combined type.

It should be noted that some uninformed skeptics (even health professionals and educators) have gone so far as to suggest that ADHD doesn't really exist and that it's nothing more than the designer disease of the late twentieth century. In reality, ADHD is a very real problem for millions of people around the world. Scientific studies have consistently identified individuals who have difficulty with concentration, impulse control, and hyperactivity. In the United States, various government departments including the National Institutes of Health, the Department of Education, the Office for Civil Rights, as well as the U.S. Congress have recognized ADHD. All of the leading medical, psychiatric, and educational groups have confirmed the existence of ADHD.

## THE BIOLOGICAL EVIDENCE

The specific evidence for a genetic influence in the development of ADHD was covered in the preceding chapter. Let's now turn our attention to the increasing substantiation for a biological expression of the genetic difference. Thanks to the development of increasingly sophisticated noninvasive techniques, the innermost workings of the human brain can be revealed. A veritable alphabet soup of imaging systems—from EEGs to PET scans, to MRIs and, more recently, fMRIs and SPECTs—are unlocking the secrets of the brain, this magnificent organ that has been called "the greatest unexplored territory in the world."

Several studies, for instance, have shown that people with ADHD have lower levels of electrical activity and decreased blood flow in the frontal brain lobes compared to non-ADHD adults and children. Other studies, principally those of Dr. Alan Zametkin and his colleagues at the NIMH, have found that people with ADHD do not use as much glucose in some regions of the brain as other people. If these parts of the brain are using less glucose, they need less oxygen and a lower blood flow. Using positron emission tomography (PET scans) the NIMH researchers found that this was happening in areas of the brain's frontal cortex. As it has long been recognized that the frontal lobes control concentration, attention span, organization, judgment, and impulses—the faculties impaired in ADHD—this finding is obviously of great significance.

Still other studies using the brain imaging tool known as magnetic resonance imaging (MRI) have discovered that children with ADHD often have slightly smaller right brains—a finding that makes sense as the right side of the brain is responsible for self-control. In pivotal research by F. Xavier Castellanos, Judith L. Rapoport, and others at the National Institutes of Health (NIH), brain scans of fifty-seven boys with ADHD, ages five to eighteen, and fifty-five non-ADHD boys were compared. These researchers found that the entire right cerebral hemisphere in ADHD boys was, on average, 5.2 percent smaller than that in non-ADHD boys.

A study in 1999 revealed that adults with ADHD have an altered metabolism of dopamine, a neurotransmitter that helps carry messages in the brain. Harvard University researchers gave a certain type of brain scan—single photon emission computer tomography (SPECT)—to six adults with ADHD and thirty others, according to their study published in *The Lancet*. This preliminary work, it is thought, could become the first objective measure of ADHD.

In effect, what all of these studies tell us is that there is a biological difference in the brains of individuals with ADHD. Children with this disorder are not just idle, naughty children who choose to be disruptive, and they are certainly not the product of poor parenting. They are individuals whose brains function differently.

## LASTING EFFECTS

At least 20 to 35 percent of children with ADHD continue with some manifestations of their disorder into adulthood. Some scientists put the figure as high as 50 percent. When you consider that many adults today were not diagnosed as children, it is likely that from 1 to 3 percent of the adult population suffers from a form of ADHD. Indeed, many adults only come to realize that they themselves have the condition when one of their children has been diagnosed.

Drs. Edward M. Hallowell and John J. Ratey have written a particularly colorful description of the adult with ADHD in their excellent book *Driven to Distraction. Recognizing and Coping with Attention Deficit Disorder from Childhood through Adulthood.* They say: "The hallmark symptoms of ADD are easy distractibility, impulsivity, and sometimes, but not always, hyperactivity or excess energy. These people are on the go, Type A personalities. Thrill seekers. High-energy-, action-oriented-, bottom-line-, gotta-run-type people. They have lots of projects going simultaneously. They're always scrambling. They procrastinate a lot and they have trouble finishing things. Their moods can be quite unstable, going from high to low in the bat of an eye for no apparent reason. They can be irritable, even rageful, especially when interrupted or when making transitions. Their memories are porous. They daydream a lot. They love high-stimulus situations. They love action and novelty."

Adults with ADHD like to go out to dinner but don't like to wait for the food to be served. When they've finished their meal and are ready to leave, they don't like waiting for others to finish. Standing in line is more tedious for them than for the rest of us, whether it's for a hot new movie or a ride at Disney World. The adult with ADHD has a work area that looks like ten years' accumulation of projects have been dumped haphazardly all over his desk. The ADHD adult has a habit of losing things he needs, such as car keys, checkbooks, wallets, and clothes.

## THE DARK SIDE OF ADHD

Many studies have followed the lives of ADHD children into adulthood and found that in general, as both children and adults, they are inclined to indulge in high-risk activities. They are more likely to smoke cigarettes, and to start smoking at an earlier age. They begin to have sex when they are younger, with more partners, and more often without protection.

One large ongoing study found that 25 to 30 percent of their ADHD group had sought treatment for sexually transmitted diseases. The study, led by eminent researcher Russell Barkley, professor of psychiatry and neurology at the University of Massachusetts Medical Center, and Mary Ellen Fisher, of the Medical College of Wisconsin, also found that ADHD women in the group had become pregnant in their late teens and early twenties. This was six years ahead of the non-ADHD comparison group. And out of forty-two births, forty-one had been born to members of the ADHD group. Sadly, about 54 percent of the ADHD participants who had had children no longer had custody of them.

Researchers Barkley and Fisher began to follow their study group—who are now in their mid- to late twenties—when they were between the ages of five and nine. They checked in with them about every five years, and their work continues to corroborate their own and other studies. By ages five to seven, Barkley says, half to two-thirds of children with ADHD are hostile and defiant. By ages ten to twelve, they run the risk of developing what psychologists call "conduct disorder"—lying, stealing, running away from home, and ultimately getting into trouble with the law. One study of hyperactive boys found that 40 percent had been arrested at least once by the age of eighteen.

ADHD children quit the education system earlier and, as a result, usually occupy lower positions on the work totem pole. As adults, says Barkley, 25 to 30 percent will experience substance abuse problems, mostly with depressants such as marijuana and alcohol. They are more likely to have traffic accidents and, in comparison with the general population, have more encounters with law enforcement and end up behind bars. One survey showed that 25 percent of male prisoners had ADHD.

ADHD is such a significant problem in the criminal justice system that the FBI's *Law Enforcement Bulletin* has addressed the issue. In June 1997, the publication carried an extensive article about the legal implications of the growing numbers of children diagnosed with ADHD. Author Sam Goldstein reported that compared to other young adults, those with ADHD "may seek excitement or stimulation, even at the expense of injuring themselves or violating the rights of others." Added Goldstein, a clinical instructor at the University of Utah School of Medicine, "Law enforcement personnel should remember that crime is not a way of life for the vast majority of persons with ADHD. However, those who engage in activities that bring them into conflict with the police generally have considerable difficulty controlling their impulses."

Furthermore, families who have children with ADHD experience increased levels of parental frustration, marital discord, and divorce and often have to bear substantial medical costs because ADHD treatment is not covered by health insurance. But there is much more to ADHD than this "dark" side. There is, fortunately, a "bright" side that has enabled many people with ADHD to become extremely successful in life.

## The Bright Side of ADHD

On the positive side, many children and adults with ADHD are bright, eager to please, and talented in a variety of ways. Some observers even regard ADHD as a gift, a hidden talent that the person with ADHD must learn how to use properly. Some believe Mozart and Edison had ADHD. A review of Mozart's life, for instance, shows that he displayed many of the hallmarks of ADHD. He was a whirlwind of energy, agitated, impatient, impulsive, easily distracted, creative, innovative, provocative, irreverent, emotionally needy, and a maverick. Edison, who may have had both ADHD and dyslexia, has been described as being "disruptive" and "misunderstood" as a child. But look what happened to him once the shackles of traditional schooling were removed. As an adult, his feverishly active mind came up with thousands of inventions that have had immense impact on our lives. What about Benjamin Franklin and Beethoven? Read their biographies and you'll discover traits commonly associated with ADHD. In the modern world, such entertainers as Whoopi Goldberg and Robin Williams, as well as such sports figures as Magic Johnson, have been described as having ADHD.

The energy and animation of a typical person with ADHD are the skills that make great performers, public speakers, and salesmen. Judyth Reichenberg-Ullman and Robert Ullman, authors of *Ritalin-Free Kids*, portray the bright side of ADHD people this way: "They can be charming, spontaneous, and fun, with a fresh moment-to-moment approach to life. People often find them more entertaining than irritating when taken in small doses. Creativity runs high in people with ADD and they often have more ideas than they can actualize effectively. They may be artistically gifted and quite sensitive."

The Ullmans go on to say, "These individuals look for the new and interesting things in life. They are inventive and often innovate new ways of doing things. These people take risks that others may fear to take, and make breakthroughs as a result. They may be dreamers, but their dreams can turn into a very gratifying and lucrative reality if they team up with others who are more grounded and follow through on their ideas."

Kate Kelly and Peggy Ramundo in *You Mean I'm Not Lazy, Stupid or Crazy?!* agree, saying, "The risk-taking behavior that gives a parent a heart attack can become a source of pride when the child grows up. She takes the big risk that puts her on the map or makes her a millionaire!" Drs. Hallowell and Ratey feel that people with ADHD can be "unusually empathic, intuitive and compassionate." And they add, "People with ADD do look out windows. They do not stay on track. They stray. But they also see new things or find new ways to see old things. They are not just the tuned-out of this world; they are also the tuned-in, often to the fresh and the new. They are often the inventors and the innovators, the movers and the doers."

One individual who has publicly acknowledged that she has ADHD is the Emmy-winning stage and screen actress Mariette Hartley. Typically, for someone of her generation, she didn't discover that she had ADHD until her daughter, Justine, was diagnosed at the age of seven. As a child herself, Mariette played the class clown to cover up her problem. "It was how I coped with life," she told the magazine *ADDitude*. Like many fellow ADHD sufferers, she struggled academically. She says that she became involved in early sexual encounters and an abusive relationship. Fortunately, she found an outlet for her energy, imagination, and talent in a successful acting career.

A classic example of apparent ADHD energy channeled in the right direction could well be renowned British entrepreneur Richard Branson, founder of the huge Virgin business empire. As a child in the United Kingdom in the 1940s it is unlikely that his behavior would have been formally diagnosed as ADHD, but he is almost a textbook case of a youngster with learning challenges. According to his official biography, he was a slow learner and at the age of eight could barely read. "High-spirited," "headstrong," and "a handful" are words used to describe the young Branson. His daredevil, rule-breaking behavior as a youth has served him well as an adult businessman. Even today his office is described as "cluttered" and his desk as "virtually invisible under a sea of papers." His hyperactivity seems to know no bounds. In December 1999 the British newspaper *The Mirror* headlined a week in the life of Richard Branson as follows: "3 international flights, 7 formal dinners, 100 interviews, 10 business meetings, 4 keynote speeches, 29 and a half hours sleep, 2 fancy dress outfits . . . and 1 Indian elephant AND THAT IS A SLOW WEEK FOR BRANSON." Accompanying the article were photographs of Branson riding an elephant, dressed as Santa Claus, and playing a tuba.

As unlikely as it could have been for Branson to be diagnosed with ADHD in 1940s Britain, it would have been out of the question for him to be prescribed a stimulant medication such as Ritalin. That's not the case today. And certainly not in the United States.

## THE RITALIN CONTROVERSY

In the United States today, the words "ADHD" and "Ritalin" are often said in the same breath. At lunchtime more than a million youngsters in schools across America stand in line for a daily ritual in which the school nurse dispenses a glass of water and a little pill. The pill is Ritalin, the most widely prescribed medication for ADHD. Critics have called Ritalin a "psychopharmacological nanny." In other words, parents and teachers are rushing to medicate kids simply as a welcome means of handling their unruly, disruptive behavior. Even a 1996 *Newsweek* cover story dubbed Ritalin "Mother's Little Helper."

Methylphenidate (Ritalin), and two other drugs, dextroamphetamine (Dexedrine), and pemoline (Cylert), have been approved by the Food and Drug Administration (FDA). The standard dose of Ritalin takes about two hours to reach maximum efficacy, and it becomes ineffective after about 4 hours. Typically, therefore, a physician will prescribe it to be taken three times a day: first thing in the morning, so that the child is alert for school; at the beginning of the lunch break, so he will again be able to focus on afternoon lessons; and then an afternoon dosage, so he will be able to concentrate on homework. Several extended release tablets, which take about four and three-quarter hours to reach peak rate and remain effective for about eight hours, have recently been approved by the FDA.

Why do Ritalin and the other drugs work? Why are they so controversial? Basically, these drugs are stimulants, chemically related to amphetamines. It doesn't seem logical that a stimulant would calm a hyperactive person. The "rational" expectation would be an increase in hyperactivity. However, put simplistically, faulty wiring in the brain is a major cause of ADHD, sparking a confusion of scrambled messages between brain cells. For reasons that are not fully understood, Ritalin enables a person to filter out the conflicting signals and focus on the task at hand. But how did stimulants come to be used for the treatment of hyperactivity? It actually began with experiments at Bradley Hospital in Providence, Rhode Island, in the late 1930s. Doctors there used a medication called Benzedrine, which is still in use today as Dexedrine, and found that giving such stimulants to hyperactive children had the unexpected effect of calming them down.

Just fifty years later, in 1988, the unanticipated result of that small test group had led to a population of half a million children being prescribed stimulants. By October 1994, one in every thirty children between the ages of five and eighteen were being prescribed Ritalin. By 1996, 1.8 million children between the ages of five and fourteen were taking the drug regularly. The trend is heading toward some 8 million children being medicated with stimulants today. It's certainly a fact that physicians in the United States prescribe five times as much Ritalin *as the rest of the world combined*. Because of its amphetaminelike structure, the Drug Enforcement Agency (DEA) classes Ritalin as a "highly addictive controlled substance" in the same category as cocaine, methadone, and methamphetamine ("speed").

Critics of the use of stimulant medications cite a 1996 DEA report stating that since 1990 there has been a 500 percent surge in prescriptions for Ritalin. Gene R. Haislip, a deputy assistant administrator at the DEA, has spoken of the agency's alarm at the "tremendous increase." He reported a 1,000 percent increase in drug abuse reports involving methylphenidate for ten- to fourteen-year-olds—equal to or exceeding that for cocaine usage. Charged Haislip, "These drugs have been overpromoted, overmarketed and oversold, resulting in profits of some $450 million annually."

Saying that in some parts of the country 15 to 20 percent of children have been prescribed Ritalin or similar stimulants, he claims there is good reason to conclude that the drugs are being used as a "quick-fix" panacea for behavioral problems. "Parents need to understand that we are talking about very potent, addictive, and abusable substances; a potency that can help in the right situation but can destroy in the wrong situation," said Haislip. "There is a legitimate place for these drugs, but we have become the only country in the world where children are prescribed such a vast quantity of stimulants that share virtually the same properties as cocaine. We must find a better balance."

One clinical trial bearing out Haislip's observations was published in the *American Journal of Public Health* in 1999. A study of two cities in the state of Virginia showed that a staggering 18 to 20 percent of white fifth-grade boys were being treated with stimulant medication. The overall rate of medication, when the entire number of subjects in the study was taken into account, was 8 to 10 percent—still considerably higher than the national average, and suggestive of regional or community variations in prescription practices.

Personally, I have not seen any evidence of widespread over-prescription of Ritalin or other stimulants (even though, of course, I would far prefer parents first take a nutritional approach). New evidence strongly refuting the overprescription charges has come from several studies. One report in the *Journal of the American Medical Association (JAMA)* in 1998 found that only 2.8 percent of all children referred to a doctor went home with a prescription for Ritalin. That study also concluded that ADHD may actually be *under*diagnosed in the general population and when compared with other countries such as Germany (9.6 percent) and New Zealand (6.7 percent). Puerto Rico, incidentally, has reported rates as high as 16.1 percent.

Peter S. Jensen, associate director for child and adolescent research at the National Institute for Mental Health, lead author on a major study published in 1999, actually says, "There is probably dramatic undertreatment with drugs." Jensen and his colleagues reported that only one in eight children with ADHD symptoms are actually prescribed medication. Analyzing survey data obtained from nearly thirteen hundred children, the Jensen team found that 5.1 percent of those diagnosed had been treated with stimulants during the previous twelve months. The study revealed that children with ADHD were more likely to receive treatment by way of mental health counseling and/or school-based interventions instead of medication. The authors' conclusion: "Medication treatments are often not used in treating ADHD children identified in the community, suggesting the need for better education of parents, physicians, and mental health professionals about the effectiveness of these treatments."

Another NIMH study in 2000 found that only half of the children positively identified with ADHD actually received care in accordance with the guidelines of the American Academy of Child and Adolescent Psychiatry. Physicians reported significant barriers to providing services for these children, including "lack of pediatric specialists, insurance obstacles, and lengthy waiting lists."

One alarming trend was revealed in a study that appeared in the *JAMA* in 2000. This study showed a dramatic increase in the prescription of psychotropic drugs to preschoolers. Over the five-year span of 1991 to 1995, researchers had examined the prescription records of more than 200,000 children ages two to four years who were enrolled on two state Medicaid programs and one health maintenance organization (HMO). In spite of the fact that Ritalin comes with a warning against its use in children under the age of six, the increase in the prescription of Ritalin rose approximately 300 percent. In total, 1.23 percent of children between the ages of two and four were being given stimulant medication.

Even more dramatic was the increase in "off-label" prescriptions for Clonidine, a medication developed to help adults with high blood pressure. Clonidine and Ritalin are being prescribed together with increasing frequency, partly to combat the insomnia associated with ADHD. Although it is prescribed only 15 to 35 percent as much as stimulants, the researchers said, "Clonidine use is particularly notable because its increased prescribing is occurring without the benefit of rigorous data to support it as safe and effective treatment for attentional disorders."

In an editorial in the same issue of *JAMA*, Joseph T. Coyle, M.D., of Harvard's Department of Psychiatry and Neuroscience, wrote, "These disturbing prescription practices suggest a growing crisis in mental health services to children and demand more thorough investigation." One month later, the U.S. government responded. At a White House press conference, First Lady Hillary Rodham Clinton announced the National Institute of Mental Health would invest $5 million researching the use of medication in treating ADHD children under the age of six. In addition, it was announced that the FDA would study the proper dosages for various types of psychiatric drugs in preschoolers and would propose requirements that manufacturers use warning labels. At the same press conference, Secretary of Health and Human Services Donna Shalala commented, "We must unlock the mysteries of children's mental health—which treatments are the most successful." So let's begin to look at other potential treatments.

## RITALIN ALTERNATIVES

Scientists are working on improved versions of Ritalin and clinical trials have already been successfully conducted on one-a-day pills that last for twelve hours. Meanwhile, one of the alternatives to Ritalin, the drug pemoline (Cylert), has become controversial as the suspected cause of acute liver failure. It was withdrawn from the U.K. market in 1997 and, although still available in the United States, the manufacturer had to issue a "Dear health care professional" letter in June 1999 announcing labeling changes. The label now advises more frequent testing of the liver function and the need to obtain written informed consent from patients and/or their parents. This came after reports of fifteen cases of acute liver failure since 1975, twelve of which resulted in deaths or liver transplantation.

As I mentioned earlier, various behavior modification techniques are often used effectively in the treatment of ADHD, and you'll find some suggestions in Chapter 9. The carrot-and-stick approach of handing out rewards for the right kind of behavior and nonphysical punishment for inappropriate behavior (time-outs, for instance) are key recommendations. Other suggested treatments—some nutritional—have become just as controversial as the use of Ritalin. Let's explore the whole issue of dietary considerations.

# DIET AND ADHD

The claim that certain foods and food additives trigger the onset of ADHD was first made in the early 1970s by Dr. Benjamin Feingold, chief emeritus of the Department of Allergy at the Kaiser Foundation Hospital and Permanente Medical Group in San Francisco. Dr. Feingold maintained that as many as 30 to 50 percent of his hyperactive patients experienced improvements when artificial colorings and flavorings were eliminated from their diet. They also benefited, he reported, from the removal of some natural chemicals such as salicylates which are found in apricots, berries, tomatoes, and other foods.

Essentially, the Feingold Diet eliminates artificial colorings (look for names such as Red 40 and Yellow 5 on labels), artificial flavorings (including vanillin, used in synthetic vanilla), artificial sweeteners (saccharin, aspartame, acesulfame-K, sucralose), and the preservatives BHA, BHT, and TBHQ. The Feingold Diet also excludes certain fruits and vegetables including apples, apricots, berries, cherries, cucumbers and pickles, currants, grapes, raisins, nectarines, oranges, peaches, peppers, plums, tangerines, and tomatoes. Also out are tea and coffee, and aspirin. (You can obtain full details of the Feingold Diet by contacting the Feingold Association—see the resource section in Chapter 11 and/or visit www.feingold.org on the Internet.)

Thousands of parents anxious for a drug-free answer began to follow Dr. Feingold's advice with many reporting improvements in the behavior of their ADHD children. Skeptics, including child development experts backed by the processed-food industry, derided his claims, which at the time did not have the benefit of controlled studies. Even today, although clinical studies have since been conducted, there is still a tendency among many health professionals to quickly dismiss a nutritional catalyst.

In November 1999, the nonprofit nutrition advocacy group Center for Science in the Public Interest (CSPI) decided it was time to address the ADHD and diet issue by producing a special report—*Diet, ADHD & Behavior*—and launching a major awareness campaign. In its "quarter-century review," the center reported that seventeen out of twenty-three double-blind studies had found evidence that *some* children's behavior significantly worsens after they consume artificial colors or certain foods such as milk or wheat.

The percentage of subjects who enjoyed improvements varied enormously from as low as 9 percent to a high of 100 percent (in one small study). One study found that children who also suffered from asthma, eczema, or hives might be particularly helped by dietary changes.(Interestingly, supplementation with long-chain polyunsaturated fatty acids often helps these conditions also. This is because an LCP deficiency makes the lining tissues of the skin, the lungs, and the stomach more permeable. As a result, materials that do not normally penetrate the body manage to get inside and cause inflammation and other allergic responses. When LCP supplements are given, the lining tissues become less permeable again. The individual then has fewer allergic reactions to the materials in the environment and the foods that were causing the problems.)

In its special report, CSPI urged parents to consider modifying their child's diet as a first means of treatment(along with behavioral therapy) before resorting to stimulant drugs. CSPI then called upon government, private agencies, and health practitioners to acknowledge the potential for diet to affect behavior. And it also urged the NIH to fund research to determine which foods and food additives provoke behavioral problems and what fraction of children is susceptible. In addition, the organization appealed for further research into the "efficacy of nutritional supplements (including fatty acids, minerals, and vitamins) in treating behavioral problems."

Said CSPI: "The drumbeat of statements from naysayers, some with vested interests, has created a conventional wisdom that diet has no effect on behavior and that Feingold's hypothesis had been disproved. Whatever the underlying reason, it is clear that many authorities appear to be unfamiliar with evidence that some children are adversely affected by diet."

There is no doubt that individual children do respond adversely to certain food components. But there is considerable doubt whether ADHD is the result of adverse reactions to specific foods, components or groups of food constituents, such as additives. There are dangers in following exclusion diets—diets that completely avoid a wide range of foods. In fact, there are dangers in avoiding even a narrow range of foods if such foods are particularly rich in nutrients—milk, for example. It makes more sense not to avoid certain foods without first discovering whether a food or particular food constituent is truly causing problems. You do this by eliminating suspect foods one at a time, and then reintroducing them one at a time. Ideally, this should be a blind test in which neither the child nor his parents are aware which foods or constituents are involved. Quite commonly, "food additives" as a group of food constituents are singled out for blame. But "food additives" may really comprise a whole host of different chemical compounds, and it would be very unusual for someone to be sensitive to all of them.

## WHAT ABOUT SUGAR?

It is commonly believed that sugar triggers hyperactivity. Obviously, the diet of many children is laden with sugar from soft drinks, breakfast cereals, and candy, as well as what is "hidden" in foods. Children (and, in fact, many adults, too) are consuming twice as much sugar as the U.S. Department of Agriculture recommends. However, not enough studies with significant numbers of subjects and of sufficient length have been done to confirm sugar as a culprit. Sugar intake may well affect some children, but nowhere near as many or as dramatically as the public thinks.

## What the Experts Say

So where does this lead us? ADHD is undoubtedly "a major public health problem." That statement was made by one of the leading experts in the United States at the end of a consensus panel convened by the National Institutes of Health. For two and a half days in November 1998 the panel considered presentations from national and international experts, as well as testimony from representatives of interested organizations and individuals. Afterwards, the panel chair, Dr. David J. Kupfer, chairman of the Department of Psychiatry at the University of Pittsburgh, painted a dismal picture of the overall state of knowledge with regard to ADHD.

Issuing an urgent call to action, he said: "There is no consistency in treatment, diagnosis or follow-up for children with ADHD. These children are subjected to a fragmented treatment system that reaches beyond health care into a wide range of social and educational support services. Its impact on individuals, families, schools, and society is profound, and it demands our immediate attention."

Recognizing that the assessment and treatment of ADHD, especially the use of psychostimulants, is as controversial as ever, the final paragraph of the panel's report is the most telling of all: "Finally, after years of clinical research and experience with ADHD, our knowledge about the cause or causes of ADHD

remains largely speculative. Consequently, we have no docu-
mented strategies for the prevention of ADHD." Saying that the
state of knowledge has been limited by short-term studies, which
have on average lasted for only three months and been primarily
focused on young, hyperactive patients, they called for more research:

- with long-term trials beyond fourteen months
- focusing on the treatment of the inattentive type of ADHD
  (which might include a higher percentage of girls)
- into ways in which both adolescents and adults are affected

They also suggested investigating treatments to improve academic performance and social skills, pointing out that current
methods such as stimulant medication merely alleviate the core
symptons.

The first study to address some of these issues was published
just over a year later in the *Archives of General Psychiatry*. The
longest-term study so far—fourteen months—it was conducted
by six independent research teams in collaboration with the National Institution of Mental Health. The researchers compared
different treatment strategies in a group of 579 children with
ADHD/combined type, ages seven to ten. The result was that children receiving a combination of medication and behavior intervention treatment, or medication alone, showed significantly
greater improvement than those receiving intensive behavioral
intervention treatment or community care without medication.

Substantial resources are now being deployed to uncover the
answers to so many vexing questions about ADHD and its treatment. Much more effort is going into the investigation of this
"epidemic" than into other disorders affecting a significant percentage of the population such as dyslexia and dyspraxia, which I
will address in the following chapters.

# CHAPTER 3

# DYSLEXIA—WHAT IT IS

*. . . dyslexic students usually have school problems, and may mistakenly be thought unintelligent, lazy or uncooperative.*

—PATRICIA VAIL, *ABOUT DYSLEXIA.*
*UNRAVELING THE MYTH*

When John tries to read, words won't stand still on the page. They appear backwards. They dance around. So much so, that the act of reading actually makes him feel sick. "When I'd sit down to read only one word stood still and the others decided to have a party. Within a matter of minutes I would become nauseous," he says. Writing was problematic, too. John would leave words out of a sentence, but when he read the sentence back to himself, he wouldn't notice they were missing. Everyone else, of course, found his comments disjointed and unintelligible. John is John O'Shea, co-author with Jenny Dalton of *Dyslexia: How Do We Learn?* In their book, he eloquently tells of his struggle with dyslexia. Among the passages that I found particularly poignant are these honest, intensely personal revelations:

- "Sometimes I felt like my head didn't belong to my body and often I thought that it had been sewn on the wrong person."
- "The thought of writing a letter was a nightmare, a thank-you note was an impossibility, and leaving a message on the door for a friend was embarrassing."
- "Skiing blind in a blizzard and going to school often feel the same to me, but skiing is a lot easier than schoolwork ever was."
- "I was catching a disease more dangerous than dyslexia; I was becoming scared to learn."

That's what having dyslexia meant to John. I've heard and read similarly graphic descriptions from others:

- "It's like being in a bicycle race, except you don't have any tires on your bike so you have to find another way to get to the finish line."
- "You get anxiety attacks, you just lose your self-esteem, you lose every feeling inside of you."
- "I think God's put my brain in upside down."

One of the most moving observations of all was reported by Sir Nicholas Monck, chairman of the British Dyslexia Association, in describing the unhappiness of a boy called Alistair, who had been motivated to write:

- "I don't want to dye . . . but I'd raver dye than go to schol tomrow."

# IN THE BEGINNING

What is dyslexia? The word "dyslexia" comes from the Greek *dys*, having difficulty with, and *lexia*, language or words. Dyslexia was first identified in the late nineteenth century when W. Pringle Morgan, a general practitioner in Sussex, England, wrote about a fourteen-year-old boy named Percy. His article, published in the *British Medical Journal*, described a boy who was "quick at games and in no way inferior to others of his age," with one major exception. Percy couldn't read. A few years later, James Hinshelwood, an eye surgeon in Glasgow, Scotland, reported in *The Lancet* cases of children suffering from what he called "word blindness." Otherwise healthy and smart, these children exhibited great difficulty reading, writing, and spelling. Hinshelwood's concern was that they be given the right kind of help, otherwise, as he wrote, "they may be treated harshly as imbeciles or incorrigibles, and either neglected or punished for a defect for which they are in no way responsible." Hinshelwood continued his studies and in 1919 a book of his articles was published, the first major treatise on the subject.

In November 1925, American neurologist Samuel T. Orton, in a now classic article, wrote about "MP," a sixteen-year-old boy from rural Iowa who "seemed bright but couldn't learn to read." Orton went on to study and describe fifteen children who shared some unusual quirky characteristics. They confused the letters *b* with *d* and *p* with *q*. Some could read better by holding pages up to a mirror. In characterizing their condition, Orton preferred to use the term "strephosymbolia," meaning "twisted symbols," rather than "word blindness." He also founded a society that is still working to help dyslexics around the world today. Formerly the Orton Dyslexia Society, it is now known as the International Dyslexia Association.

In addition, Orton hypothesized that difficulties with learning to read and write were the result of faulty brain functioning, stemming from the failure of one brain hemisphere to establish dominance over the other. Orton turned out to be remarkably prescient in identifying many of the hallmarks of dyslexia that have stood the test of time, for there is much more to dyslexia than confusing *p*'s and *b*'s or numbers such as 6 and 9.

Some of those hallmarks pinpointed by Orton include:

- The ability to read text just as easily, or more easily, upside down or in a mirror
- Stuttering, other speech impediments, and/or slowness in acquiring the ability to talk
- A high occurrence of left-handedness or ambidexterity
- Clumsiness
- Extremely bad spelling
- Family history of dyslexia

Dyslexia seems to be rooted in a person's inability to translate letters into sounds, a serious difficulty in distinguishing phonemes, the smallest sounds that make up speech. The English language contains a total of forty-four such sounds. The word "cat," for example, is made up of three phonemes or sounds: kuh, aah, and tuh. Most people readily understand that, and it becomes an unconscious part of reading.

Leading dyslexia researcher Dr. Sally Shaywitz of Yale University puts it like this. To learn to read all children must discover that:

1. spoken words can be broken down into smaller units of sound
2. letters on the page represent these sounds
3. written words have the same number and sequence of sounds heard in the spoken word

# Dyslexia—How It Is Diagnosed

Different criteria for diagnosing dyslexia are used from country to country, and there's often dispute, even within a country, as to what exactly constitutes a diagnosis. Experts make an evaluation based on reviewing a child's history, through personal observations of the child, and by performing psychometric (psychological measurement) tests. Standardized tests of reading and spelling are usually conducted along with tests of ability in other areas.

The most commonly used test is the Wechsler Intelligence Scale for Children (Revised), known as WISC-R. There is a similar test for adults, the Wechsler Adult Intelligence Scale (WAIS). These scales test three measures of ability: Verbal IQ, Performance IQ, and Full Scale IQ. The Verbal IQ assesses how effectively information presented auditorily is memorized and used for problem solving and concept formation. The Performance IQ tests how information is used for the same purposes when presented visually. The Full Scale IQ is derived from a combination of the other two scales, and gives a general indication of all-round ability. Dyslexics usually have a higher Performance IQ than Verbal IQ. They also have recognized patterns of scores in the following subtests, which make up the Verbal and Performance IQs.

| Verbal Subtests | Performance Subtests |
|---|---|
| Information | Picture completion |
| Similarities | Picture arrangement |
| Arithmetic | Block design |
| Vocabulary | Object assembly |
| Comprehension | Coding |
| Digit span | |

Typically for the dyslexic, the weakest scores will be for arithmetic, coding, information, and digit span—often referred to as the ACID profile. There are some other measures of performance that are derived from the subtest scores, such as spatial ability, conceptual ability, and sequencing ability. Quite typically, dyslexics score the highest in spatial ability, then conceptual ability, and worst in sequencing ability. A diagnosis of dyslexia is made when an individual with poor reading and spelling ability, which cannot be attributed to low IQ or inadequate educational opportunity, has these IQ and subtest profiles.

The Wechsler tests are performed by fully trained educational psychologists who are skilled in their administration and interpretation. However, much simpler checklists like the one given at the end of this chapter can help you identify dyslexia in a family member, and can be helpful as a preliminary to full testing.

How prevalent is dyslexia? Some researchers put the number of dyslexics in the United States as high as 20 percent, and although it used to be thought that boys considerably outnumbered girls, recent research at Yale University indicates that just as many girls suffer from reading disabilities. The National Institute of Child and Human Development (NICHD) suggests that up to 17 percent of children have a reading disorder that could be called dyslexia (many of whom are not identified as such in schools).

The National Center for Learning Disabilities (NCLD) agrees, saying that at least 17 to 20 percent of children have a significant reading disability. The NCLD states: "Unfortunately, the rate of reading failure and illiteracy are unacceptably high in the United States. Over 40 percent of fourth-grade students performed below basic levels on the National Assessment of Educational Progress (NAEP) in both 1994 and 1998. Over 10 percent of fourth-grade children could not even participate in the NAEP due to severe reading difficulties."

The NCLD goes on to say: "It is also noteworthy that large numbers of school-age children from all social classes, races and ethnic groups have significant difficulties learning to read. Because reading is so critical to success in our society, reading failure constitutes not only an educational problem but also rises to the level of a major public health problem."

## THE BIOLOGY OF DYSLEXIA

But what causes dyslexia? How are dyslexics different? Clues have emerged, both from autopsies of the brains of dyslexics and through brain scans. Dr. Albert Galaburda and colleagues at Harvard Medical School found a major difference in the brains of ten dyslexics that they autopsied and compared to brains of non-dyslexics. In most people, the left side of an area of the brain, the plenum temporale, is always larger than the right. In dyslexics, both sides of the brain were equal (or, in some instances, the right side was larger).

Recent technological advances in brain imaging that allow in-depth studies of how the brain works have confirmed these observations. In addition, it now appears that there are anomalies in the structure and function of those parts of the brain connecting the right and left hemispheres (the corpus callosum) and in the area of the brain involved in coordination and balance (the cerebellum). Dyslexic individuals also exhibit a level of disorganization and reduced sensitivity in the magnocellular pathway within the brain, the large-cell superhighway responsible for the accurate high-speed perception of rapidly changing stimuli such as movement and sound variation.

## MORE THAN WORDS

The inability to decipher sentences is only one of the difficulties people with dyslexia encounter. A recent study in *The Lancet* suggests that dyslexics also have problems in learning skills unrelated to words and language.

Researchers led by Roderick I. Nicolson of the University of Sheffield, England, used the brain scanning technique positron emission tomography (PET) to compare the brain activity of six adult dyslexics with six nondyslexics. Participants were asked to perform a sequence of finger movements that they had learned earlier, as well as a similar exercise that they were taught during the study itself. The researchers noted significant differences in blood flow in the cerebellar cortex, the outer layer of the cerebellum, the part of the brain responsible for the coordination of voluntary movement, balance, and muscle tone and also associated with learning skills. The average increase in cerebral blood flow in the two tests was 7.5 percent for the normal individuals versus just 1.4 percent for the dyslexics. An increase of blood flow in an area of the brain is an indication that it is working harder.

## EARLY CLUES

Dyslexia is often not formally identified until a child goes to school and encounters difficulty learning to read and write in comparison to her classmates. Frequently, a child may be nine years old before an official diagnosis is made. But there were many clues much earlier in the child's life.

The preschool child might persistently jumble words. She may ask to eat "bizgetti" or "hang-a-bers," and say "callapitter" instead of "caterpillar." She might substitute words, for example, saying "lampshade" when she meant to say "lamppost." She may have difficulty learning nursery rhymes and rhyming words such as cat, sat, mat. From a seemingly obvious group of items she might not be able to select the odd one out, such as dog, pig, house, and cow. She may forget the words for familiar everyday objects, such as table, chair, and house. The dyslexic preschooler will probably not master the art of speaking clearly until later than expected. She will enjoy having a book read to her but will not display any interest in the letters or words on the page. She will also, most likely, share some characteristics with dyspraxic children. She may be inattentive. She may trip, bump into objects, or fall over much more than most children her age. She may be uncoordinated, having difficulty in the usual childhood pursuits of hopping and skipping, as well as catching, throwing, and kicking a ball. She may find it hard to clap in time to a simple rhythm. She may also be inattentive and find it hard to remember and follow directions.

In the first years of school, difficulties with reading and spelling become very apparent. She will put letters the wrong way round—the well-known confusion of *b* and *d*, *p* and *q*, *w* and *m*, *h* and *n*, and other similar letters. She will probably have corresponding problems with some numerals. She may leave letters out of words or put them in the wrong order. She may read "saw" for "was," "God" for "dog," and "on" for "no." She may also have great difficulty reading aloud. In conversation or in class, dyslexics often have trouble finding the words they need as quickly as they need them. They're often disorganized and messy.

Dyslexics often have an awful sense of time. They don't know whether five, ten, or twenty minutes have lapsed since last asking their parents the time. They have difficulty differentiating between the future and the past. She may ask, for instance, "Is yesterday the day after tomorrow?" Dyslexics tend to confuse directional words such as "up" and "down," "left" and "right," "in" and "out." When asked to read, she might ask, "Where does the book start?"

Sequences such as days of the week, numbers, and months of the year also tend to throw her. The sequence of the alphabet is especially challenging, and creates basic difficulties such as finding words in a dictionary or names in a telephone directory.

Many dyslexic children have difficulty with arithmetic, particularly when it comes to learning multiplication tables. She will probably need to count using her fingers or make marks on paper to work out simple calculations, while other children can do it in their heads. Once early problems with calculation are overcome, however, she may go on to be highly successful at math, as it is a subject more broadly concerned with the relationship between things in shape, size, quantity, and space. Reading a musical score is nigh on impossible, yet the dyslexic may have a good musical ear and be a talented performer. Many dyslexics have good and bad days, for no obvious reason. She may perform superbly on one test and do terribly on the next. She may recognize a word in one sentence, and then stumble over it in the following sentence. And yet, for a child who seems challenged in so many ways, she will often surprise you with how smart she can be.

There are other similarities with dyspraxic children: She may have difficulty dressing herself—tying shoelaces and doing up buttons, for example. She may have a persistent language delay and immature uses of tenses and sentence construction. She may have a lisp or speech impediment. As the dyslexic child reaches high school, difficulties will persist. As a result, she will likely be lacking in confidence and self-esteem. She will almost certainly continue to struggle with reading and spelling. She will stumble over long words. As John O'Shea expressed it, she may find that words on the page are "having a party," or that the text often disappears, shooting off into a "page wormhole." She may continue to confuse places, times, and dates. Instructions and telephone numbers will need to be repeated. Planning and writing essays will be extremely arduous tasks.

She will most likely have poor handwriting, and still fail to grasp the basic rules of punctuation and capitalization. A classic example is the handwriting and spelling of one famous dyslexic, Thomas Alva Edison. They were so bad that, even as an adult, his correspondence looked like that of a child. It's very striking in a letter that he wrote to his mother when he was nineteen years old:

> *Dear Mother—Started the Store several weeks. I have growed considerably. I don't liik much like a Boy now— Hows all the folk did you receive a Box of Books from Memphis that he promised to send them—languages. You son Al.*

Edison's abilities showed themselves in other ways. Dyslexics (like many children with ADHD) tend to daydream excessively and have vivid imaginations. No wonder Edison was such a brilliant inventor! Albert Einstein, *Time* magazine's Person of the Century, who reputedly suffered from both dyslexia and ADHD, was another great dreamer. He once received a school report stating: "Albert is a lazy boy who never tries to do his work. He daydreams all the time." Throughout school, Einstein repeatedly received bad marks for his reading and writing. For Edison and Einstein, reading and writing remained a lifelong struggle, as it is for so many lesser-known dyslexics today. But dyslexics are frequently adept at recruiting others to help them overcome their handicap:

- General George Patton, a dyslexic, matriculated at West Point with the help of other students whom he paid to read his textbooks to him.
- Winston Churchill, another dyslexic, got through school by having his mother read to him. He "wrote" his famous speeches and award-winning books mostly by dictating to a stream of secretaries.

- Hans Christian Andersen's publisher could make no sense out of his offerings until a friend of Andersen's "translated" his writing.

Most dyslexics work hard at hiding their condition, often going to extreme lengths to maintain an elaborate pretense. As adults, they're reluctant to discard the protective shield they have built around themselves. Look at their handicap by thinking of the road to literacy as being like a long-distance car ride. Most of us take the freeway—the shortest, fastest, most direct route. But for a dyslexic, it's as if a major accident has blocked all the lanes. Result: They have to exit and take a long, meandering detour. They get there eventually; it's just a longer, more circuitous journey.

Says Barbara Guyer, author of *The Pretenders*: "Having reading problems is different from any other problem a person might be challenged with. If you can't draw or sing or play a musical instrument, if you can't balance a checkbook, or if you fail in an attempt to master a computer program, or the elements of biology, you can probably laugh about it. But if you can't read words on paper, you will typically feel ashamed and try to hide this gap from everyone you meet. Each time you tell a lie to mask your problem your self-esteem goes down another notch." Worse still, the ridicule and stigma attached to dyslexia take their toll in more tragic ways. Trudy Carlson, author of *Learning Disabilities*, says that people with dyslexia are three times more likely to suffer from depression than are people without a learning disability.

## ACADEMIC "UGLY DUCKLINGS"

Like Edison and Einstein (and some say Leonardo da Vinci), many dyslexics display extraordinary talents and become highly successful in different walks of life. Many are creative-thinkers, risk-takers, people with grit and determination, entrepreneurs, and pioneers, people who push the envelope.

One modern example is Jack Horner, the revolutionary dinosaur researcher whose theories forced paleontologists to rethink the established wisdom. Horner consistently failed exams at the University of Montana because of his dyslexia. "Back in the days when I was growing up, nobody knew what dyslexia was . . . so everybody thought you were lazy or stupid or both. And I didn't think I was but I wasn't sure," the adult Horner told the *Chronicle of Higher Education.* Horner did have remarkable determination: "I had a lot of drive, and if somebody told me I was stupid, that usually helped. It really helped me take a lot more risks. For somebody that everybody thinks is going to grow up to pump gas, you can take all the risks you want. Because if you fail, it doesn't matter."

Actor Tom Cruise, another dyslexic, says that for him it began in kindergarten: "I was forced to write with my right hand when I wanted to use my left. I began to reverse letters, and reading became so difficult. I was always ashamed." The Cruise family (his real name is Thomas Cruise Mapother IV) moved frequently because of his father's job as an engineer. Cruise attended fifteen different schools. "That made the problem worse," he recalled in a *Parade* magazine interview. "With my reading difficulties, I'd never catch up. But people would excuse me: 'He's the new kid. We'll just help him through this year.' " Cruise's mother, who had studied to become a teacher of special education, recognized the symptoms of dyslexia and gave him extra tutoring. Added Cruise, "I had to train myself to focus my attention. I became very visual and learned how to create mental images in order to comprehend what I read."

Pioneering stockbroker, Charles Schwab, who spearheaded the introduction of discount stock buying, credits his battle with dyslexia for helping him develop other talents—the ability to envision, to anticipate, to be a creative problem-solver. Craig

McGraw, developer of the cellular telephone industry, says that his ability to think in a nonlinear fashion is also connected to his dyslexia. Weighty written documents are hard for him to absorb. Instead, he sits back and thinks about the big picture. No wonder a *Fortune* magazine cover described him as a "dyslexic visionary."

Patricia Vail, a nationally recognized authority on dyslexia, learning disabilities, and the education of the gifted child, describes such luminaries as having been "academic ugly ducklings." (Ironic, since Hans Christian Andersen, author of *The Ugly Duckling*, was also dyslexic.) Nevertheless, it's harder in today's society for someone with dyslexia to rise above the crowd. Getting ahead in the late twentieth/early twenty-first centuries is more dependent than ever on passing exams and getting "letters after one's name"—achievements that usually require written skills.

We often hear family histories of grandparents, for instance, who could not read yet built successful businesses or farms. Today, in spite of notable exceptions, the nonliterate individual is not so easily absorbed into the workforce. As Thomas West, author of *In the Mind's Eye*, says: "Today, with extensive academic preparation required in almost every field (using traditional verbal modes of instruction and testing), it seems quite clear that many highly talented dyslexics are being excluded by groups and disciplines that could greatly profit from their vision, enthusiasm, perceptiveness, creativity and originality." In fact, in real-life situations such as hands-on training, sports, and the arts, dyslexics often learn faster than the average person.

## THE COSBY FAMILY

Some educators, psychologists, and teachers don't approve of putting labels on children. The result is that there's often a failure to identify a child's problem. But the diagnosis of dyslexia is often a cause for relief, even celebration, after years of an individual feeling just plain dumb. Such was the case with Bill Cosby's son, Ennis, whose untimely death at the hands of a gunman made headlines in early 1998. Ennis has been quoted as saying, "The happiest day of my life was when I found out I was dyslexic."

Bill Cosby vividly remembers that day. As he told the nation on ABC's "Good Morning America," "When we got the word that Ennis was dyslexic a cheer went up." That was because they knew he was intelligent and capable of doing better. Since a root cause had been identified, they could begin to find out *how* he learned. Added Mr. Cosby, who has since made it a mission to enlighten the public about what it means to be dyslexic, "If you don't know about dyslexia, you think that the person has something wrong, is dumb, is not as bright."

Ennis Cosby's dyslexia was not recognized until his sophomore year at college. The result was dramatic. Once he mastered some effective learning strategies his grade point average went from a 2.3 to a 3.5. In his case, those strategies meant learning to visualize words in patterns instead of memorizing letters. The identification of Ennis's dyslexia was as if a lightbulb had been turned on in his head, giving him a wider appreciation of the problem. Quickly, he realized that his uncle, Bill Cosby's brother Russell, displayed some of the same symptoms. At age fifty-two, Russell was persuaded by Ennis to go to Landmark College, the country's only accredited college specifically for students with learning disabilities, where Ennis's condition had been spotted. Russell discovered that he, too, is dyslexic. It's not surprising, of course, since, as we've discussed, dyslexia runs in families, especially those with particularly talented or creative individuals.

Says teacher Carolyn Olivier, author of *Learning to Learn*, who helped launch a learning program at Landmark, "The biggest problem dyslexics face is misunderstanding, and that teacher looking at that student is going to think that perhaps he's not smart, perhaps he's lazy, unmotivated, not paying attention." That's what Russell Cosby encountered as a youth. As he told an audience at the Harvard Graduate School of Education, "The kids were saying I was stupid. The neighbors were saying I was dumb. The school system said I was slow. So my mother took me to a psychiatrist who said, 'He'll grow out of it—I promise you.' Well, I never did." Two years after enrolling at Landmark and discovering he was reading at a third-grade level, Russell says, "Now if you saw me you'd think I was going for my Ph.D. I love it. I enjoy it."

Ennis Cosby was in his sophomore year before he discovered he was dyslexic. His uncle, Russell Cosby, was fifty-two years old when he was diagnosed. Today, it should not be so late in anyone's life before dyslexia is diagnosed. Following is a simple checklist that anyone can use to assess dyslexia.

## THE RICHARDSON DYSLEXIA SYMPTOM INTERVIEW CHECKLIST

A way of assessing whether someone has dyslexia has been devised by Dr. Alex Richardson of Oxford University. It is conducted as an interview so that, if necessary, additional information can be captured. Dr. Richardson is currently collecting data to validate terms and categories of the checklist, and to quantify the relationships with other tests for dyslexia. But as you will see from the ratings list at the end, dyslexics can be clearly identified. In this checklist, interviewees are asked to rate the applicability of each item to themselves as:

0 (not at all)
1 (just a little)
2 (quite a lot)
3 (very much)

## Visual Symptoms Experienced During Reading

When you try to read, how much are you bothered by the following?

Headaches or eye strain
Losing your place on a page
Particular problems with small, crowded print
"Double vision"—that is, letters and words splitting in two
Print becoming blurred or out of focus (even with glasses)
Letters or words moving around on the page or board
Letters or words moving "in and out" of the page or board
A distorted (stretched or twisted) appearance to the print
Glare or discomfort from reading in bright light
The appearance of a fringe, halo, or aura around words
Problems or discomfort from reading a computer screen*
Difficulty reading subtitles on TV or at the movies*

## Auditory Perceptual Problems with Language

When listening to language, how much are you bothered by the following?

Difficulty following and understanding very rapid speech
Problems decoding speech against background noise
    (music, traffic, machinery, or other environmental
    sounds)
Difficulty following speech when you can't see the speaker's
    face or expressions
A particular problem in concentrating when more than one
    person is talking—for example, in a crowded room or
    at a party

*These questions used for adults only.

Difficulty hearing clearly in a large (but quiet) lecture or
school hall

Trouble understanding the speaker if he or she has a strong
accent

### Difficulties with Spoken Language

When using language, how much are you bothered by the
following?

Word-find difficulties—for example, in rapid naming or
recall

Using too few words when explaining something (not
giving enough detail or elaboration)

A tendency to give long, complicated, or roundabout
explanations (too much detail, not enough structure)

Talking very fast, with a tendency to ramble on

Talking very slowly and carefully, but often missing the
chance to join in or say what you want as a result

Stuttering or getting tongue-tied

Pronunciation problems, especially with multisyllabic
words

### Motor Coordination Problems

Rate any problems you may have in the following areas.

General clumsiness (tripping, knocking things over)

Difficulty with balance (riding a bicycle, climbing, reaching,
or leaning)

Problems in catching or hitting a ball at speed (tennis,
badminton, racquetball, squash, softball)

Problems with fine motor coordination (threading a needle,

sewing, sorting beads, making models, skilled
carpentry, etc.)
Difficulty acquiring the skill to perform a new set of
movements (learning to drive, driving a different car,
learning a new keyboard routine, learning a sport, or
dance sequence, etc.)

## How Do You Rate?

The complete scoring system has not yet been established for all
age groups. However, an assessment of adult dyslexia can be made
depending upon the following scores.

Visual symptoms when reading: There is a strong chance of
someone being dyslexic if they score over twelve. On average,
nondyslexics score three in this subscale.

Auditory perceptual problems with language: There is a
strong chance of someone being dyslexic if they score over seven.
On average, nondyslexics score three in the subscale.

Difficulties with spoken language: There is a strong chance of
someone being dyslexic if they score over nine. On average,
nondyslexics score three in this subscale.

Motor coordination problems: There is a strong chance
of someone being dyslexic if they score over four. On average,
nondyslexics score two in this subscale.

A high score in any one of these four categories is a good indication that someone has dyslexia. Obviously, if someone scores
high in all of the subscales she is much more likely to be dyslexic.
In these circumstances, it would be wise to consult an educational
psychologist for a full assessment. It is interesting to note that one
of the measures for dyslexia is a problem with motor coordination, a condition shared with children who have dyspraxia, the
subject of the next chapter.

# CHAPTER 4

# DYSPRAXIA—THE "UNKNOWN" DISORDER

*Without intervention, a dyspraxic child grows into a dyspraxic adult.*
—MADELEINE PORTWOOD, CHAIRPERSON OF THE
EDUCATION COMMITTEE OF THE DYSPRAXIA
FOUNDATION, UNITED KINGDOM

Peter is accident-prone, clumsy, and uncoordinated. In school and at home, at work and at play, his days usually consist of a series of mishaps and confusion. He tends to bump into furniture and people; to fall down, to drop things. He's generally gawky and awkward. He has a poor sense of balance, which became obvious when he tried to learn how to ride a bike. For some reason, he just can't seem to catch a ball or throw one with any degree of precision. Invariably, if he tries to kick a ball, it doesn't go where he wants it to go. And he's just as likely to trip over the ball, anyway.

Team sports are definitely not his thing. The other kids, of course, have recognized his limitations, and Peter always experiences the indignity of being the last selected for a team. Getting changed to play sports brings its own set of challenges. Peter is slower than the other kids. Sometimes he will put both legs inside one pant leg or put his shirt on backwards and amble out of the changing room long after the others are already at play. His shoelaces may still be loose, his shirttail hanging out, buttons undone. Peter compensates by playing the fool. He's the class clown. He'll cover up his inadequacies by pretending that he's really just horsing around. He finds it difficult to make friends and rather than play with children his own age, he'll play on his own or with older or younger children.

In the schoolroom, Peter's handwriting and drawing skills are well below the standard. He has a hard time using scissors, drawing with crayons, wielding a paintbrush, and manipulating puzzles and construction blocks. In fact, any kind of manipulation, including such seemingly straightforward tasks as turning a doorknob, utilizing silverware, and screwing lids on and off containers, presents great difficulty. His teacher always needs to repeat information. Organizing his thoughts well enough to write a story is a daunting task. Often, he'll forget to take his books to school.

Socially, Peter also has problems. Visitors may throw him into turmoil, he's uneasy in a crowd, he doesn't like to be touched—even resisting his mother's comforting embrace—and he suffers motion sickness. He has an intense dislike of various textures; he hates to touch sand and slime and certain foods. Particular smells and sounds can irritate him. Emotionally, Peter is an enigma. Sometimes he reacts excessively, other times he doesn't react at all. Often it's an inappropriate reaction, either way. His emotional pendulum swings higher and lower than that of most people. Having his hair washed, taking a shower, brushing teeth and hair—these normal everyday personal care tasks are an ordeal for him. He likes routine. Unexpected changes cause great distress and lead to crying, screaming, throwing punches, or hiding. New and unpredictable situations completely throw him. It's more difficult for him to cope with a new house, a new teacher, and a new anything than it is for other children.

Peter, quite literally, doesn't know what day of the week it is or that Thursday comes after Wednesday. The time of year in relation to the months is baffling to him. He doesn't understand which towns are nearest to his home. He may have difficulty putting a series of thoughts together. Yet, if anything, he is of above average intelligence for his age and is frustrated by his inability to display it. Peter is dyspraxic. Not all dyspraxic children, of course, have all of these symptoms, but many display a number of them to varying degrees.

## DYSPRAXIA—THE OFFICIAL DIAGNOSIS

Dyspraxia, also known as developmental coordination disorder, the term endorsed by the American Psychiatric Association in 1994, affects 5 to 10 percent of children, up to 2 percent severely. Some researchers have put the number even higher—as high as 20 percent. At least four times more boys than girls are affected (some researchers estimate as many as seven times), although girls, when they are affected, are usually more severely disabled.

The American Psychiatric Association's *DSM-IV* lists five criteria upon which to base a diagnosis:

1. A marked impairment in the development of motor coordination.
2. The impairment significantly interferes with academic performance or daily living activities.
3. The coordination problems are not the result of a general medical condition, such as cerebral palsy, hemiplegia, or muscular dystrophy.

4. It is not a pervasive developmental disorder.
5. If developmental delay is evident, the motor difficulties are greater than those seen in normal children.

Associated features listed by the manual include phonological disorder, expressive language disorder, and mixed receptive-expressive language disorder. The Dyspraxia Foundation puts it more simply: "Dyspraxia is an impairment or immaturity of the organization of movement. Associated with this there may be problems of language, perception and thought." One of the best tools for assessing impairment in the development of motor co-ordination (poor movement skills) is the ABC Movement Assessment Battery developed by Henderson and Sugden. This test battery consists of two parts. First, there is a checklist, completed by an adult familiar with the child, that asks questions about the child's movements in relation to the environment. Second, there are a series of tests of movement skills like catching and throwing balls, balance skills, and fine motor skills like handwriting.

Says Dr. Helene Polatajko, professor and chair of occupational therapy at the University of Western Ontario, Canada: "A substantial body of information attests to the legitimacy of the disability as a worldwide phenomenon with a prevalence greater than 5 percent of the child population. There is now strong scientific evidence that the motor problems of these children persist at least into adolescence, that they are more likely to demonstrate poor social competence, academic problems, low self-esteem, and that they are less likely to be physically fit or participate voluntarily in motor activities."

Dyspraxia is the "poor relation" of this trio of learning disorders that I have investigated. Awareness of the condition, though increasing, is far less than that for ADHD and dyslexia, especially in the United States. In addition, the variety of symptoms and the ability of bright children to disguise their problems mean that many cases may go undiagnosed. Dyspraxia has, however, been recognized since the beginning of the twentieth century when it was first described as "congenital maladroitness." In 1937, Dr. Samuel Orton declared it to be one of the six most common developmental disorders, and in 1975, eminent dyspraxia researcher and neurologist Dr. Sasson S. Gubbay gave it the label "clumsy child syndrome."

Over the years other terminology has been used: developmental awkwardness, sensorimotor dysfunction, minimal brain dysfunction, and motor sequencing disorder. The World Health Organization (WHO) currently uses the term "specific developmental disorder of motor function." Whatever the label, dyspraxia undoubtedly causes major disruptions in the lives of those it afflicts and of their families and friends. Dyspraxia is a disorder of *praxis*, a Greek word meaning "doing, acting, deed, practice." Praxis includes both knowing what to do and how to do it—doing without thinking. It is what links brain and behavior, enabling us to think and effectively act upon those thoughts. First one has an idea (ideation), then it's necessary to know how to implement that idea (motor planning), and then to actually be able to carry it out (execution). It's the capacity to function in new and innovative ways.

Says Judy Davies, author of *Planning to Move, Moving to Plan*, and a member of the Dyspraxia Support Group of New Zealand: "Somewhere along the line the messages are not getting through, are not producing the right result. Praxis is inconsistently failing. Inconsistently, because yesterday or this morning the message may have been getting through, and the child may have been able to perform the task, but now he can't, now the plan has been lost somewhere. It may turn up again at another time or the child may have to relearn the plan, skill or task."

## LACK OF RECOGNITION

I believe a lot of dyspraxic children are not being identified early enough, either by the education system or by doctors. Parents often feel that there is something wrong with their child at an early age, but well-meaning health and education professionals comfort them by saying that he's "just a late developer." Parents usually bow to the greater knowledge of the expert only to be proven right—later than they would have liked. This "lost" time could have been spent on intervention programs and the introduction of nutritional supplementation.

In a U.K. survey of 450 members of the Dyspraxia Foundation, most parents said they were aware that their child had a problem by the age of three, but, on average, an official diagnosis was not made until the child was six and a half. Only a quarter of dyspraxic children are recognized as having the problem when they start school, and four out of five schools think the child will "grow out of it." More than a third of the schools even blamed the children's conduct on "bad parenting."

Worse still, less than 2 percent of family doctors in the United Kingdom even consider that a child might have dyspraxia. The country's health visitors—nurses who make home visits and usually a parent's chief contact with the medical community—are even less inclined. Only 1 percent of them are likely to contemplate a diagnosis of dyspraxia. The same survey revealed that half of the children's teachers had never even heard of the condition!

The same situation exists around the world. Many doctors have not yet become fully educated about dyspraxia and are just not aware that it is an acknowledged medical condition. They see it, but they really don't know what it's about or what to do about it. Unfortunately, the consequences of letting dyspraxia go unnoticed and untreated can be severe. Like children with ADHD, dyspraxics' sheer frustration with their condition can foster negative social behavior and frequent confrontations with law enforcement, resulting in incarceration. This was highlighted when noted dyspraxia researcher Madeleine Portwood tested juveniles in a young offenders institution. Portwood, senior educational psychologist with Durham County Council in the United Kingdom, found that a staggering 61 percent of the offenders were dyspraxic, but none of them had ever been diagnosed.

Dyspraxia can confidently be identified before the school years begin; in fact, some problems can be recognized in the first three years of life, even at birth. A baby later identified as dyspraxic may have been unusually irritable, allergic to milk, and colicky. Establishing regular sleep habits may have been difficult and he may not have responded well to his mother's efforts to comfort him. The dyspraxic child is slow to achieve many of the standard childhood milestones of sitting up, talking, walking (they usually bypass the crawling stage), and toilet training. At nursery school, the dyspraxic youngster may seem aggressive because of his inadequate communication skills. Mothers sometimes describe their toddlers as "all arms and legs," who keep falling over and bumping into furniture. Temper tantrums and night terrors often occur.

Between the ages of three and five the dyspraxic child will be a bundle of energy, swinging arms, tapping feet, and clapping (although he'll have difficulty tapping and clapping in time to music). He won't be able to sit still for more than a few minutes. He may find it hard to concentrate on performing various tasks. He can be forgetful and disorganized, anxious, sensitive to touch, and easily excitable. His hands may flap when running or jumping, and he won't be able to catch or throw a ball. Pedaling a tricycle will not come easy. He will avoid construction-type toys such as Legos. And his eating habits will continue to be uncoordinated. Food and drink fly everywhere.

When it comes to fine motor skills such as handling a pencil or a pair of scissors, the dyspraxic child will be frustrated. He probably won't be able to draw an identifiable man, as he'll be struggling to decide where to place "real" arms and legs. Unlike most children of this age, he doesn't display the same delight in imaginative play or "dressing up." In fact, he'll be far behind his peers in learning to put his regular clothes on.

## The Years of Challenge

It's when a dyspraxic child starts school that he encounters the most monumental challenges. This is the time when his mother leaves him at the school door and he's expected to stand on his own two feet, to fend for himself. This is the time when his clumsiness will make him stand out from the other children, when he'll be regarded as an oddball, and more likely than not be singled out for criticism by both teachers and classmates.

He will be poor at physical activities. Throw a ball to a dyspraxic child and you'll note that he's standing in an awkward posture, legs apart, licking his lips, anxious. He may fall down before the ball reaches him or totally miss it, as if the ball mysteriously evaded his hands. He doesn't like to "cross the midline"—that is, he won't like trying to catch a ball with both hands to one side of his body. Similarly, you will notice that the dyspraxic child will not work with his books in front of him; he will push a notebook to the side to write in it. His handwriting will be poor and he will have a hard time copying, tracing, or writing within lines. He will find it difficult to copy things from the blackboard. He will be unable to understand instructions and have difficulty expressing himself. The dyspraxic child often spends more time doing his homework than other children, and, sadly, with much less to show for it.

Says Dr. Sasson Gubbay: "The problems are greatest in the earlier school years when there is an increasing expectation for the child to attend to his own personal needs. The continual reprimands for untidy handwriting or drawings and bungling efforts in team ball games are demoralizing. The child may recourse to inventing illness or other indispositions in order to avoid ridicule by his peers or he may resort to clownish behavior to create the impression he is not really trying his best." Neralie Cocks, author of *Watch Me, I Can Do It!*, agrees that the typical school curriculum imposes great pressure on the dyspraxic child. She says, "Life can be stressful for children with motor difficulties because so much of the primary school day revolves around motor-based activities, both in the classroom and in the playground."

That was certainly the case for eight-year-old Jake, the second son of musician and singer Sting. A typical dyspraxic child, at school he was constantly losing things. His classmates noticed that he always took longer changing into his gym clothes, and that he had difficulty tying his shoelaces. Not surprisingly, the other children tormented and bullied him. His teacher's repeated criticism for being lazy and demands that he try harder didn't help.

"Of course, Jake's self-esteem plummeted. From being a boisterous, lively bundle of energy, Jake was transformed into an insecure worrywart," his mother, Trudie Styler, wrote in a *Harper's Bazaar* article. "He could see that other kids could do with ease things that were hard for him, and he didn't understand why. He would say, 'There's something wrong with my brain; I know there is.'" Trudie, a filmmaker, actress, and environmental activist, went on, "Sting and I both felt guilty we had unwittingly chosen a school that was damaging our child, but we also felt very angry. Our little boy had become unrecognizable. He was hostile, aggressive, and afraid of everything."

After Trudie and Sting consulted a battery of understanding teachers and psychologists, the clinical neuropsychologist at London's renowned Great Ormond Street Children's Hospital finally diagnosed dyspraxia. Since then, Jake has been attending a school where the teachers have a good understanding of his condition and Jake, aware of the ways in which he is different, is developing a growing confidence.

The dyspraxic child's ineptness at physical activities—whether sports, manual hobbies, dancing, or music—generally encourages passive pursuits such as reading or watching television. Consequently, the youngster tends to become isolated, as there is less motivation to make friends. Dyspraxics have huge problems because everyday life is so frustrating for them. They may be no good at writing and no good at sports, so it's not just academically, not just in the classroom, it's also playground interaction where they literally fall down.

Life can be extremely tiring for dyspraxic children as they have to work harder than other children at seemingly ordinary activities. "They have to approach each action as if it were a first-time try and concentrate when other children are moving easily, apparently without thought," says Christine Macintyre, author of *Dyspraxia in the Early Years.* "Children with coordination difficulties have problems in synchronizing their movements so that they can appear 'all fingers and thumbs,' clutching at air as the ball sails past, having to stop walking or running before they place the dish on the table, or not being able to move out of the way as they close the door. They can't do two types of task at the same time. The children don't easily 'get it together,' and tend to have stilted rather than flowing movement patterns. 'Awkward' and 'jerky' are common descriptors of the way children with coordination difficulties move."

Fortunately, dyspraxia is a problem largely confined to childhood as long as children receive therapy. These children can and do improve, but they do not simply outgrow it without help. The small proportion of children who do take their clumsiness with them into adult life can usually manage the condition, especially as there is less pressure to conform to arbitrary norms. As adults, there is less demand on skills that are part of a child's existence such as playing ball games and balancing. But those dyspraxics whose conditions persist into adulthood may, of course, not only still be clumsy and uncoordinated, but they may also display little sense of direction and have difficulty driving a car or riding a bike. They may also find it hard to follow instructions and pay attention to what others are saying, another example of the overlap between ADHD, dyslexia, and dyspraxia. They may be forgetful and socially awkward, inappropriately butting in on conversations, for instance.

As you will discover, nutritional supplementation with long-chain polyunsaturated fatty acids can help children with dyspraxia as well as children with ADHD and dyslexia. But before we turn to the specific research validating LCP supplementation for children with these disorders, let's review the importance of fat in the human diet.

# THE SCIENCE

# CHAPTER 5

# THE FATS OF LIFE

*Ultimately, fat is as essential to your health as vitamins,*
*minerals, antioxidants, carbohydrates, and protein.*
*Good fat is good food.*
—ARTEMIS P. SIMOPOULOS, M.D., FORMER CHAIR OF
THE NUTRITION COORDINATING COMMITTEE,
NATIONAL INSTITUTES OF HEALTH

Fat is good for you! Fat is essential for life. Fat impacts every function of your body from the beating of your heart to the nanosecond communications within your central nervous system. In fact, you may be surprised to learn that your brain is 60 percent fat. Yet for many years fat's reputation as a dietary component has been unfairly tarnished. It is true, of course, that excess dietary fat, just as excess calories from any source, unhappily turns into unwanted body fat, obesity, and the ill health associated with it. On the other hand, insufficient dietary fat may interfere with growth. Deficiency of some fats may even foster a mélange of behavior problems, including depression.

The essential fatty acids are as important to your physical

health as vitamins, minerals, trace elements, electrolytes, protein, and carbohydrates. In this chapter, however, I am going to show you why these shorter-chain EFAs and, to a much greater extent, their longer-chain polyunsaturated fatty acid (LCP) derivatives are even more critical for brain health. In particular, I will reveal just how important they are in alleviating the symptoms of learning disorders such as ADHD, dyslexia, and dyspraxia. Looking at the science helps explain the respective merits of EFAs and LCPs.

## THE ESSENTIAL FATS

First, let's consider the two essential fatty acids—linoleic acid (LA) and alpha-linolenic acid (ALA)—that are, indeed, essential for life, as they are vitally involved in the proper functioning of every cell, tissue, and organ in the human body. Like vitamins, they cannot be produced by the body. They have to come from the food we eat. LA is found in seed oils such as sunflower, safflower, corn, and sesame. ALA is found in dark leafy vegetables, flaxseed oil, and rapeseed oil. The human body cannot make LA from ALA (and vice versa). Therefore, we need to get both from food.

Both LA and ALA have eighteen carbon atoms in their chainlike molecules. These have to be converted into longer-chain fatty acids with twenty or twenty-two carbon atoms in order to fulfill some of their vital functions in the body. As you can see from the adjacent illustrations, the molecules also have unsaturated bonds, another important chemical feature.

Sometimes called double bonds, unsaturated bonds are between some of the carbon atoms. LA has two unsaturated bonds; ALA has three unsaturated bonds. The position of the first unsaturated bond in the chain is biologically important, and is named either "n" or "omega." There are two main families of fats

### Linoleic acid (LA)

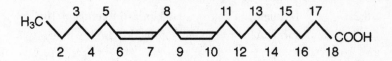

### Alpha-linolenic acid (ALA)

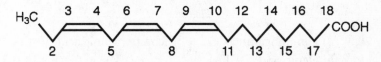

with more than one double bond. They are the n-3 or omega-3 family and the n-6 or omega-6 family. The name comes from the fact that the first double bond is either three or six carbon atoms from the end of the chain. The essential fatty acids, ALA and LA, are the first members of the omega-3 and omega-6 families.

Just as ALA and LA are transformed in the body by making the chains longer, they are also transformed by adding more unsaturated bonds. In the omega-6 family, LA—with two double bonds—is converted to arachidonic acid (AA) and adrenic acid (AdrA), which both have four double bonds, and is eventually converted into omega-6 docosapentaenoic acid (DPA), with five double bonds. At the head of the omega-3 family, ALA, which starts with three double bonds, is converted by several steps into eicosapentaenoic acid (EPA) with five double bonds, and then docosahexaenoic acid (DHA) with six.

The conversion of one fatty acid to another involves processes of desaturation and elongation controlled by enzymes. The conversion process can be slowed by many lifestyle factors, including typical Western diets rich in trans fatty acids, stress, viral

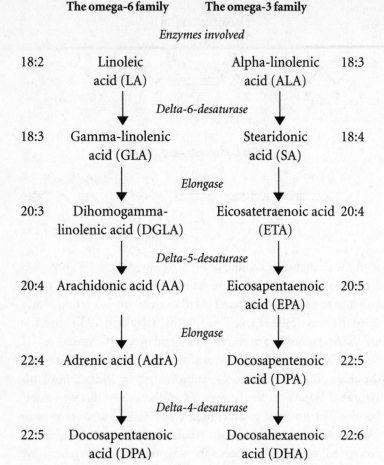

**The omega-6 family**　　　**The omega-3 family**

*Enzymes involved*

| 18:2 | Linoleic acid (LA) | Alpha-linolenic acid (ALA) | 18:3 |

*Delta-6-desaturase*

| 18:3 | Gamma-linolenic acid (GLA) | Stearidonic acid (SA) | 18:4 |

*Elongase*

| 20:3 | Dihomogamma-linolenic acid (DGLA) | Eicosatetraenoic acid (ETA) | 20:4 |

*Delta-5-desaturase*

| 20:4 | Arachidonic acid (AA) | Eicosapentaenoic acid (EPA) | 20:5 |

*Elongase*

| 22:4 | Adrenic acid (AdrA) | Docosapentenoic acid (DPA) | 22:5 |

*Delta-4-desaturase*

| 22:5 | Docosapentaenoic acid (DPA) | Docosahexaenoic acid (DHA) | 22:6 |

Scientific Note: This is a somewhat simplistic representation, but it is suitable to demonstrate the conversion process. There is evidence that in the omega-6 chain, the conversion of adrenic acid (AdrA) to docosapentaenoic acid (DPA) may well be more complicated than illustrated. Similarly, in the omega-3 chain, the conversion of DPA to docosahexaenoic acid (DHA) may also be more involved than is shown here. In this book I am referring to LA and ALA as essential fatty acids. When fatty acids of both the omega-6 and omega-3 families have more than twenty carbon atoms, they are referred to as long-chain polyunsaturated fatty acids.

infections, too much alcohol, and various illnesses. As you will discover later, one of the key problems that children with ADHD, dyslexia, and dyspraxia appear to have is in converting the eighteen-carbon essential fatty acids into the effective longer-chain derivatives.

A chart summarizing the conversion of the omega-6 and omega-3 essential fatty acids into longer chains with more unsaturated fatty acids is given above.

Long-chain polyunsaturated fatty acids (LCPs) play an integral part in the formation of the brain's complex network of 100 billion cells. We're all "fat heads," as there's actually a greater percentage of fat in the brain than in any other organ. Half of this fat is LCPs, the building blocks of membranes in the brain. DHA is the most abundant omega-3 LCP in the brain, and AA and AdrA are the most abundant omega-6 LCPs.

Don't confuse DHA with DHEA which has gained widespread publicity for its purported antiaging properties and is totally different from DHA. DHEA (dehydroepiandrosterone) is the most abundant steroid hormone in the body. It is involved in the production of testosterone, estrogen, progesterone, and corticosterone. As the body's DHEA stores decline with age, some experts have maintained that putting it back into the body in later life, in the form of supplements, will have many health benefits. *DHA is quite different; it's an LCP that your brain can't live without.*

We will be delving further into the role of the LCPs in brain development, but it is important to note that there is a substantial amount of evidence proving that omega-3 fatty acids deliver a wide range of health benefits. These include relief of arthritic symptoms such as stiffness, pain, and inflammation; reducing women's risk of breast cancer; and preventing the painful intestinal ailment known as Crohn's disease. Omega-3 supplementation has also been shown to prevent and ease emphysema, chronic bronchitis, and asthma attacks.

A truly dramatic illustration of the fact that some fats are beneficial to health and not harmful (as popularly believed) came through an examination of the eating habits of the Greenland Eskimos. These people ate a lot of fat, mostly from the meat of the fish, seals, and whales they caught. Yet they had a very low rate of heart disease. Similar studies investigating the eating habits of Norwegians and Japanese fishermen—two groups also known for eating plenty of cold-water marine fish—showed similar results.

It was quite a puzzle until scientists subsequently discovered it was because of *the kind of* fat that they were eating. The Eskimos, the Norwegians, and the Japanese fishermen were getting omega-3 LCPs, which had quite the opposite effect to that attributed to saturated fats and cholesterol. Studies have since demonstrated that LCPs both help prevent heart attacks *and* their recurrence. One study found that men who regularly ate fatty fish were 42 percent less likely to die from a heart attack than men who did not eat such fish. Another study with a twenty-year follow-up showed that there were 50 percent fewer deaths among men who began consuming at least 30 grams of fish per day after a heart attack. And a major review of seventeen controlled trials showed that supplementation with an average of 3 grams per day of omega-3 LCPs led to a significant reduction in blood pressure. This beneficial effect occurred relatively quickly—thirteen of the studies were less than three months long.

So, the omega-3 LCPs are most definitely good fats. Their impact on general health is momentous—even though the population as a whole may not yet have gotten the message. Considering the bad reputation of "fat" in the modern Western world, it may be hard to comprehend the critical role that the good fats have played in the evolution of mankind. Let's make a journey back in time, therefore, to explore the very origins of the human race and give the LCPs, the long-chain polyunsaturated fatty acids, the recognition they deserve.

## LCPs and the Dawn of Mankind

For approximately 4 million years our ancestors roamed the planet hunting and gathering their food. Everything they ate grew or lived in the wild—from the fruit, nuts, and herbs they collected to the animals they stalked and killed. During this period almost 100 percent of our genetic structure evolved. But what led to the massive brainpower of modern man, an intelligence that eclipses all other creatures? Highly respected researchers such as C. Leigh Broadhurst, Stephen C. Cunnane, and Michael A. Crawford have argued that humankind's superior brainpower is the *direct* result of the abundance of LCPs in the food supply of our Paleolithic ancestors.

Evidence clearly indicates that man evolved in the East African Rift Valley, a unique geological environment with many enormous freshwater lakes. These waters provided an abundance of fish, crustaceans, mollusks, and algae rich in the long-chain polyunsaturated fatty acids EPA, DHA, and AA, which we now know to be essential nutrition for the brain. It's highly probable that early man *directly* secured his fill of these nutrients by capturing and eating fish and other marine life. In addition, it's extremely likely that he obtained this critical nutrition *indirectly* by eating other creatures who also dined on the marine life—birds, small mammals, reptiles, and amphibians. Even more certainly, he obtained further supplies of LCPs by eating the eggs of these creatures.

Researchers Broadhurst, Cunnane, and Crawford have developed a colorful picture of early man satisfying his hunger by grabbing or trapping fish and crustaceans by hand, and smashing the shells of mollusks. Obviously, these were somewhat unsophisticated activities, but ironically they yielded a bountiful catch of brain-boosting nutrition. That's because the fat profile of tropical and subtropical freshwater fish and other aquatic species have a DHA:AA ratio closer to that in brain phospholipids—the bricks and mortar of nerve cell membranes—than any other food source. (*Phospho* means that the substance contains the mineral phosphorus. *Lipid* means that it contains fat molecules. Phospholipid, therefore, simply means a substance that has both phosphorus and fat.)

Early man thrived, most likely, on this readily available marine life so profuse in LCPs. In a 1998 article in the *British Journal of Nutrition*, the team of Broadhurst, Cunnane, and Crawford envisioned a scenario in which hominids scavenged fish and/or fished opportunistically, which helped increase intelligence enough for them to fish more often and more successfully. They wrote, "In order to sustain the rapid expansion of the cerebral cortex, generation after generation of early Homo must have had access to sources of abundant, balanced PUFA [polyunsaturated fatty acids], most probably in the form of AA and DHA at a ratio of about 1:1."

We know with some assurance the eating habits that not only helped the human species evolve but also ignited the mental prowess of mankind. For tens of thousands of years this hunter-gatherer diet was the mainstay of human existence. The first significant change came with the advent of the Agricultural Revolution some fifteen thousand years ago. The cultivation of crops and the raising of domestic animals were the beginning of a fundamental and radical shift in our diet that led to the consumption of vegetable oils, dairy products, grains, and refined sugars.

Evolutionary nutrition expert Boyd Eaton, M.D., of Emory University, puts it into perspective this way: "Americans think of bread and milk as quintessentially 'natural' foods. . . . However, from the standpoint of genetically determined human biology, these foods are Johnny-come-latelies." It is just in the last one hundred years, however, that the most extraordinary change has

taken place in the human diet. It is a change that has had a profound impact on our health, and may well be revealed to be a pre-
dominant factor in the dramatic increase in learning disorders.

## A CENTURY OF CHANGE

Exactly what has changed in the last one hundred years? The most
striking difference is the amazing decrease in the consumption of
the all-important omega-3 LCPs and a corresponding increase in
consumption of omega-6 LCPs from vegetable oil. Researchers believe that about 60 percent of Americans are now deficient in
omega-3 LCPs and about 20 percent of them have so little that test
methods can hardly detect any in their blood. How has such a dramatic imbalance occurred over the course of a human lifespan?

There are three key reasons: (1) a major change in food
manufacturing processes, (2) a major change in our diet, and (3)
a major change in breast-feeding habits.

### Food Manufacturing

The major change in food manufacturing processes has been la-
beled "The Horror of Hydrogenation." It created what are known
as trans fatty acids. How and why did we create such fats? The
"culprit" is the food industry, which about one hundred years ago
invented hydrogenation, the method of turning liquid vegetable
oil into solid margarine or cooking fats. Hydrogenation was introduced for several valid reasons. First, the customer at the time
preferred solid fats. You need solid fats to spread on bread and you
cannot use liquid fats (oils) for baking pastries, cookies, and
cakes. Second, the polyunsaturated vegetable oils are unstable;
they readily react with oxygen in the air and become rancid.

Rancid fats taste bad and are not good for health. So, for reasons of convenience, cooking, safety, shelf life, and flavor, hydrogenation became routine.

Today we devour substantial quantities of hydrogenated and partially hydrogenated vegetable oils, not just in margarine and cooking fats but in a cornucopia of snacks, convenience foods, and baked goods. Today, almost 10 percent of the fat we consume is trans fat—that's between 10 and 15 grams per person per day. One hundred years ago we consumed hardly any!

Such twentieth-century alchemy is commercially understandable, but it has unfortunate consequences in terms of health. The trans fatty acids formed by hydrogenation act differently in the body than other fats do. They not only seem to impair the production of the beneficial LCPs, but they have also been implicated in an increased risk of cardiovascular disease, diabetes, and possibly cancer. Furthermore, it is no coincidence that the prevalence of learning disorders seem to be worse in more highly developed countries, the very countries with the increased consumption of hydrogenated fats.

The food manufacturing industry, however, is not solely responsible for the downturn in our consumption of LCPs. Not to be outdone, the livestock industry began to fatten up farm-raised animals with large amounts of corn and soybean meal that contain omega-6 fatty acids, but little or no omega-3 fatty acids. The chicken, beef, and pork that now finds its way onto our dinner tables has higher omega-6 fatty acids and much less omega-3 fatty acids than in past times. Even today's farmed fish tends to have less omega-3 fatty acids because of the food upon which the fish are raised. As far-fetched as it may sound, in one study of farmed fish it was discovered that they weren't getting the LCPs they needed from the food chain. To enable them to see better so they could find and capture the other food they needed, they had to be supplemented with LCPs. Strange, but true!

Animals grazing in the wild—elk, deer, and bison, for instance—have as much as five times more omega-3 fat content than domesticated animals. This is because the plants they eat provide them with shorter-chain omega-3s that their bodies can slowly convert to the longer-chain polyunsaturated fatty acids EPA and DHA. Similarly, free-range cows, chickens, and other animals have much higher levels of omega-3s because they also eat lots of green leafy vegetables. Some chicken and eggs provide omega-3 LCPs when poultry are fed with fishmeal or algae-enriched feed containing DHA.

## Our Destructive Diet

Over the course of the twentieth century we have chosen to eat less of the foods naturally rich in DHA—cold-water fish such as tuna, salmon, and mackerel, and organ meat. According to U.S. Department of Agriculture statistics, among American who eat fish, the daily intake of DHA went down from 168 milligrams in 1950 to 92 milligrams in 1994. Among Americans who don't eat fish, the consumption of DHA dropped even more dramatically, from 100 milligrams a day to 34 milligrams. Also during the last one hundred years we have begun to eat more and more of the foods ladened with trans fatty acids that block the production of DHA.

Imagine what happens if membranes in your brain need a DHA refill, but you haven't been eating food containing DHA—such as tuna and salmon—or even enough of the precursor short-chain omega-3 fatty acid ALA. Instead, like most Americans, you've been eating French fries, doughnuts, potato chips, and other food loaded with omega-6 and trans fats (almost half of the fat in some bags of potato chips is trans fat). If there isn't enough DHA, the body's first choice as fat for the membranes is the omega-6 long-chain fatty acid DPA, and it substitutes with that.

But your brain needs the omega-3 LCPs. If it doesn't get it, it has no choice but to make the most similar fat it can—the omega-6 DPA—from the fat that you've force-fed it. But the omega-6 DPA molecules are shaped differently from DHA. Your brain reluctantly takes the wrong fat and the result is akin to building a wall with bricks that don't fit, or trying to bake a cake without a major ingredient. The chemistry of the membranes around and within the nerve cells changes. The messages between brain cells get scrambled and interrupted. Nothing works as efficiently.

Ridiculously, our fear of fat has even led manufacturers to produce low-fat tuna, and fat-free salmon patties, stripping the fish of its most prized nutritional gift. Noted nutrition expert Artemis P. Simopoulos, M.D., former chair of the Nutrition Co-ordinating Committee of the National Institutes of Health, is aghast at such meddling. With more than a touch of sarcasm, she says, "Eating fat-free salmon makes as much nutritional sense as buying carrots that have been stripped of their beta-carotene or oranges that have been hybridized to be low in vitamin C."

We talk about "modern civilization," but we don't eat as many brain-healthy foods as cavemen did. The diet of the hunter-gatherers would have had an omega-6 to omega-3 ratio of between 1:1 and 1:5. Today, the ratio in the Western world is completely reversed: We eat a shocking ten to twelve times more omega-6 fatty acids than omega-3s.

What this means is that today's common diet is completely out of synch with our genetic imprint. The balance of foods that we now eat is totally at odds with hundreds of thousands of years of evolution. While the difference in the genetic makeup of modern man compared to that of our Paleolithic ancestors is minuscule, the kind of food that we now "hunt and gather" from supermarket shelves is vastly different.

On top of all this, a simplistic "low-fat, high-fiber" dietary message has been drummed into the public consciousness by well-meaning nutritionists and the media. It has become so ingrained that many parents have adopted it as the dietary standard for their children, even for infants. But nutrient requirements for the growing child are so very different. I once made a very careful presentation on this subject at a national conference in the United Kingdom. As soon as I highlighted a point by saying that it might be better for a child to eat a chocolate bar than an apple, the journalists rushed out of the room to file their stories. They had an easy headline! But there was a serious motive behind the simplistic allusion. The point I was making was that chocolate is good for the growing child because it provides more energy as well as iron and copper—nutrients that she needs. Unfortunately, all the antifat propaganda has misled parents. They don't seem to realize that growing children frequently need more energy from sugar, fat, and carbohydrates than adults do, and that some foods so rich in the much-despised fat provide other important nutrients as well.

This became very evident when I organized a study at the University of Surrey with my colleague Dr. Jane Morgan and a graduate student, Alison Redfern, in which we asked one thousand mothers what they were feeding their kids. To our great concern, we discovered that mothers who were weaning their children onto solids—children under one year of age—were avoiding fat. They were giving their babies lots of fruits and vegetable purees, which are obviously valuable sources of nutrients, but they're not enough. These infants were not getting the fat or the calories or certain nutrients that they need, such as iron and zinc.

Further proof came from a separate study, which reviewed the British government's National Food Survey, an annual report on the diets of seven thousand households. This revealed that babies in the United Kingdom in the 1990s were consuming

20 percent fewer calories than babies a quarter century earlier. Our survey of parents with infants between three months and one year of age showed that 83 percent of them favored high-fiber foods for their babies and an astonishing 88 percent believed that a *low* fat intake was important. Wrong! Right for adults, maybe, but completely the opposite requirement for babies. Too much fiber fills a baby up too quickly, and low-fat foods can impair growth and development.

So-called healthy-eating guidelines suggesting that we eat more fruit and vegetables and avoid fat—guidelines really designed for weight control in adults—have somehow become the gold standard for the entire population. Some babies, therefore, are being placed on diets that deprive them of vital nutrients— such as long-chain polyunsaturated fatty acids—that their growing bodies desperately need. More than four out of five mothers have been trying to put their children on a "nursery starvation diet" of vegetables and fruit purees and low-fat yogurts rather than traditional foods. Fortunately, not many succeed because hungry babies intuitively know what they really need, so they cry and demand more food.

The fact that 5 percent of children admitted to pediatric hospitals in the United Kingdom are admitted because of malnutrition or failure to thrive is extremely worrying. Most alarming, as we shall see, is the overwhelming evidence that newborns are often deprived of the LCPs that are critical for their mental and physical well-being, literally from the moment of conception. This is not only because of the mother's eating habits but also because they are less likely to be breast-fed.

## Changes in Breast-Feeding Habits

In fact, there has definitely been an overall decline in breast-feeding leading to a serious deficiency of omega-3 fatty acids in many people. A fully breast-fed baby gets all the nourishment she needs from her mother's milk (as long as the mother is well-nourished). All of the protein, vitamins, minerals, carbohydrates, and, yes, essential fatty acids and long-chain polyunsaturated fatty acids are freely and readily available. Nature does know best.

But let's step back a few months. In the womb, the fetus is totally dependent upon the mother for nourishment. During the first few weeks of conception, before most women even realize they are pregnant, the young embryo is undergoing her most active period of brain cell division. Some 70 percent of the dietary energy fed by the mother to the fetus is dedicated to meeting the demands of the fetus brain's prodigious rate of growth.

Just how demanding is the fetus? How much of a drain is there on a mother's nutritional stores? A University of Minnesota study by Dr. Ralph Holman and colleagues found that during pregnancy the level of omega-3 fatty acids in the blood of mothers-to-be dropped considerably when compared with non-pregnant women. The study continued for six weeks after birth and the fatty acid deficit persisted. DHA was found to be only 35 percent of its prepregnancy level. A similar study led by Dr. Monique Al produced similar results, and also discovered that the decline of DHA became worse with subsequent pregnancies.

It has actually been demonstrated recently that the mother's brain shrinks by roughly 3 percent during the nine months of pregnancy. Why? The most likely explanation is the growing need of the fetus for AA and DHA. The needs of the mother's brain for these LCPs is subservient to the needs of the fetus. Any LCPs made

## BRAIN FOOD

The rapidly growing baby brain has a huge demand for fatty acids.

ARACHIDONIC ACID (AA): A long-chain omega-6 fatty acid, AA is necessary to achieve normal birth weight and circumference of the baby's head, as well as cardio-vascular development.

ADRENIC ACID (AdrA): A long-chain omega-6 fatty acid made from AA in the body. Few foods provide AdrA, so it is important to take enough of the precursor AA.

DOCOSAHEXAENOIC ACID (DHA): A long-chain omega-3 fatty acid, DHA is critical for the healthy development of the brain, central nervous system, and vision.

by the mother's tissues or provided from food may well go to the fetus first. Growing another brain takes its toll on the mother—and may be one of the reasons for the memory loss that some associate with pregnancy.

After birth, for the first four months of life, and maybe even for as long as six months, the baby looks to her mother's breast for nearly all of the nourishment she needs. And not just for the development of good physical health, for the development, too, of good mental health. And improved brain power.

## INCREASING IQ

Are breast-fed babies really brainier than formula-fed babies? The answer is a resounding yes! Many studies have shown that breast-fed infants have statistically higher IQ and improved visual perception compared to formula-fed infants. Some research has also shown that the longer the period of breast-feeding, the better the mental performance. A major analysis of twenty studies published in September 1999 showed that breast-fed infants scored three to five IQ points higher than their formula-fed counterparts. The review, which appeared in the *American Journal of Clinical Nutrition,* took all possible variables into account, including the education and socioeconomic status of the mother. Its conclusion: Breast milk nutrition was solely responsible for the cognitive advantages.

But is this just a short-term benefit? Not at all. A study of three hundred children, all born prematurely, demonstrated that those who had been given breast milk were a staggering eight IQ points ahead of those who had received formula not containing LCPs. The children were eight years old when their IQ was measured, according to a Cambridge University study headed by Professor Alan Lucas and published in *The Lancet* in 1992. More recently, a study of more than one thousand eighteen-year-olds proved even longer-lasting academic benefits from breast-feeding. New Zealand researchers L. John Horwood and David M. Fergusson reported in a 1998 issue of *Pediatrics* that breast-fed babies were 38 percent more likely to grow up to successfully graduate from high school than their formula-fed counterparts. What's the difference? In particular, it's the LCP known as DHA. Several studies have demonstrated that breast-fed term infants have higher levels of DHA in the brain than formula-fed infants, indicating that elevated DHA in the diet correlates with elevated DHA in the brain.

Subsequent research has gone on to show benefits in a direct comparison of infant formula with and without the LCPs. In a trial at the University of Dundee in Scotland, forty-four term infants, for the first four months of their lives, were given either a formula supplemented with LCPs or formula without the LCPs, but containing the precursor essential fatty acids LA and ALA. At the age of ten months they were given a test that involved uncovering and retrieving a hidden toy. The infants who had received the LCP supplement did significantly better, suggesting that beneficial effects persist beyond the actual period of supplementation, says the study published in *The Lancet* in 1998.

A more recent American study, published in March 2000, compared the development of infants who were fed either formula supplemented with LCPs or ordinary commercial formula without LCPs. Those getting the LCPs did significantly better. In the study, conducted by Eileen Birch and her group at Retina Foundation of the Southwest in Dallas, and published in *Developmental Medicine & Child Neurology*, fifty-six newborns were divided into three groups. For the first four months of life the groups were fed different formula. A control group received a commercial formula with nothing added. One test group was given formula supplemented with DHA, while the third group was given formula containing both DHA and AA. At the end of the four-month period all the children began to receive regular commercial formula.

When the children reached the age of eighteen months they were tested on the Bayley Scales of Infant Development, a standard test used to gauge physical and mental progress of infants. A score of 100 is considered the national average for mental development. The group of infants who received the DHA/AA combination formula scored 105.6—virtually identical to the score of a separate group of babies in another study who were breast-fed only. The DHA group scored 102 and the group that received the commercial formula lagged behind with a score of 98. The children in the study are going to be tested again at the ages of four and nine to determine if the enhanced early brain development continues in later school performance.

Other studies have shown that full-term infants who have no DHA in their diet for the first year after birth have poorer vision than babies receiving DHA. The difference between the two groups is "equivalent to one line on an eye chart."

## THE MISSING LINK

Citing the importance of DHA in the neurological development of children, Horwood and Fergusson recommended the need to "develop improved infant formulas with properties more similar to those of human breast milk that may lead to improved developmental outcomes in children." This is the crux of the problem as DHA is a major constituent of breast milk but is not always found in manufactured formula. In fact, until recently, in the United States, in stark contrast to about sixty other countries around the world, no infant formula contained any DHA. American babies were deprived of this crucial LCP, whereas American puppies and kittens were not. DHA is now being added to one company's milk replacer formulae for puppies and kittens!

Because formula-fed babies in the United States "are deprived of this essential building block," there are "incalculable quality-of-life issues," says Frank A. Oski, M.D., former chairman of pediatrics at the Johns Hopkins University School of Medicine. Studies indicate, he says, that "for every year of delay, more than two million formula-fed full-term babies born annually in the United States may experience a disadvantage of three to six IQ points compared with breast-fed full-term babies." The difference, adds Professor Oski, is even greater for infants with low weight at birth.

Researchers Broadhurst, Cunnane, and Crawford, who have traced the evolutionary importance of DHA, agree. They say, "Long-chain polyunsaturated fatty acid deficiency at any stage of fetal and/or infant development can result in irreversible failure to accomplish specific components of brain growth. There is good evidence today that lack of abundant, balanced DHA and AA in utero and infancy leads to lower intelligence quotient and visual acuity and in the longer term contributes to clinical depression and attention deficit hyperactivity disorder."

Growing demand for the inclusion of DHA in infant formula is now coming from doctors throughout the United States. Pregnant Physicians for DHA, a resource group of the DHA Information center at Rockefeller University in New York, claims over one thousand physician members. "Optimal brain development requires the DHA and AA provided by breast milk," they say, urging that both of these LCPs be incorporated into all U.S. infant formulas.

Barbara Levine, Ph.D., chief of nutrition at New York Hospital–Cornell Medical Center, strongly supports this position, adding, "DHA deficiency may also be involved in postpartum depression and may play a role in other emotional/ mental problems." The need to obtain adequate LCPs, says Dr. Levine, goes beyond pregnancy and babyhood: "DHA is as important throughout the rest of life as it is at birth. According to studies, children without adequate DHA may be more likely to develop behavioral and learning problems, such as ADHD."

Referring to the debate over whether infant formula in the United States should be supplemented with LCPs, Dr. Leo Galland, director of the Foundation for Integrated Medicine in New York, says, "Questions have been raised such as 'Is it necessary?' and 'Is it safe?' but mostly it's a question of politics rather than science. There are a lot of egos involved. Maybe it's the cost—and manufacturers certainly don't like to change their formulas when they have a product selling tens of millions of units a year. You don't want to change unless there are compelling commercial reasons."

The FDA has the matter under review and is expected to issue new regulations for U.S. formula makers in the near future. But across the Atlantic, the wisdom of adding LCPs was formally recognized almost ten years ago. The European Society for Pediatric Gastroenterology and Nutrition recommended in 1991 that formulas for premature babies be supplemented to give them as much DHA and AA as breast-fed babies. Since then, a host of influential international organizations have recommended that formula for full-term healthy babies be supplemented. Among them, the British Nutrition Foundation, the United Nations/World Health Organization (WHO) Expert Committee on Fats and Oils in Human Nutrition, and the International Society for the Study of Fatty Acids and Lipids.

In the United States, Americans spend a staggering $3 billion a year on infant formula when their babies could be getting better nutrition—*free*. In fact, 38 percent of American mothers never even try breast-feeding. And despite strong recommendations from the American Academy of Pediatrics and the American Dietetic Association that mothers should nurse their babies for at least a year, a mere 15 percent do so. That's one of the lowest rates in the world.

The problem is partly the result of misinformation. Many new moms interviewed by researchers at the University of Minnesota, like the mothers in my U.K. survey, actually doubted that they could produce enough milk to keep their babies healthy. Moreover, there are more women than ever in the workforce. Many of them are returning to work soon after giving birth, an obvious obstacle to their ability to breast-feed. In fact, nearly half of the mothers in the Minnesota study named their jobs as an impediment to breast-feeding. It is not an insurmountable impediment, however, as the mother's expressed breast milk can easily be saved in a bottle and given by whoever is taking care of the baby while the mother is at work.

## THE DHA DILEMMA

Even when American mothers do breast-feed, there's still no guarantee that their children are getting the nutrition they need. In the United States today, even the best-intentioned mother dutifully breast-feeding for a year or longer may still not be providing her baby with sufficient DHA. The shocking truth is that DHA levels in the breast milk of American women are among the lowest in the world and typically deliver just one-half to two-thirds of the minimum amount of DHA recommended for infant formula by the World Health Organization and the U.N. Food and Agriculture Organization. Breast milk of the modern American mother just does not have as rich a natural supply of LCPs as her grandmothers' milk.

The reason? We're back to the issue of diet. Many women do not enjoy a diet abundant in DHA and instead eat a variety of manufactured foods loaded with trans fats. Because they are not getting enough LCPs in their diet there's every possibility that their children are being malnourished in the womb. If the mother is deprived of DHA, the embryo is certainly deprived, too. And just imagine what happens when a mother has a second child in quick succession to the first. Quite often it's noted that the younger sibling struggles because the demands of the previous pregnancy have left the mother without sufficient LCPs. A deficiency of LCPs has also been linked to depression. Could this be why so many women suffer depression after childbirth? Leading NIH researchers Drs. Joseph Hibbeln and Norman Salem certainly think so. They say, "This relative maternal depletion of

DHA may be one of the complex factors leading to increased risk of depression in women of childbearing age and in postpartum periods."

## IN SUMMARY

Let's review where we have gone wrong. We're eating far too much of some fats—the omega-6 fats and hydrogenated and trans fats—in our manufactured foods. We're not eating enough of the omega-3 essential fatty acids and omega-3 LCPs that the brain needs to function properly. So, not only are we getting less of the good fats in our diet, we're also greatly diminishing the value of the good fats that we do consume. It's an amazing double-barreled shotgun blast of damage to brain development.

Some women do not have enough DHA in their system to transfer to the baby either in utero or by breast-feeding after birth. Further, many women elect to bottle-feed instead of breast-feed, which, in the United States, means that the newborn infant gets none of the vital DHA at all. All of this can exacerbate any LCP deficiency that may already be present in genetically predisposed individuals. For those individuals who cannot convert the shorter-chain EFAs into the longer-chain polyunsaturated fatty acids, the result may well be a breakdown in communication between brain cells, leading to the development of learning disorders such as ADHD, dyslexia, and dyspraxia as well as other neurobiological problems.

If we continue to eat the way we've been eating, there's little doubt that more and more children will suffer learning disorders of one kind or another. So, what can we do? There is a wealth of research and recommendation with regard to protein and other nutritional requirements for body growth. In comparison, there is surprisingly little research and recommendation highlighting the importance of fats and brain growth. A flurry of research published as the twentieth century came to a close prompted Michael A. Schmidt, author of *Smart Fats*, to say, "Our increasing knowledge of the way in which fat affects the brain . . . may turn out to be one of the most important discoveries of the century."

Schmidt may well be right. In the next chapter we'll look at some of the new research, especially as it applies to learning disorders. Then we will show you how you can immediately begin to take advantage of the latest scientific knowledge by adding enough omega-3 LCPs to your diet to bring your body back in line with man's genetic nutritional requirements.

# CHAPTER 6

# THE BREAKTHROUGH RESEARCH

*The simple news that Nature told*
—EMILY DICKINSON

A complex three-dimensional jigsaw puzzle—that's how I like to think of the many-faceted aspects of research leading to the exciting discovery that supplementation with long-chain polyunsaturated fatty acids (LCPs) can help learning disorders. There are many pieces to this particular puzzle that have fallen into place through innovative studies at institutions around the world. The first pieces, as outlined in the previous chapter, were the discovery of the important role of LCPs for a healthy brain, as well as for a healthy body. Evidence of the special value of the LCPs in mother's milk filled in another eye-opening piece of the puzzle.

All of this was familiar to me. I had studied it and taught it during my career of more than thirty years at the University of Surrey in the United Kingdom. In fact, I've had a longtime interest in infant nutrition as well as other public health issues such as obesity. In particular, I've been concerned about the fact that there is such a focus on obesity when undernutrition is also a major problem, even in affluent societies, and especially for babies, as you discovered in the previous chapter.

Personal considerations stepped into my professional world, however, when my son, James, was diagnosed as dyslexic. This family challenge heightened my interest in this subject. At the outset, I was not deliberately looking for a nutritional solution. As a family, we first went along the well-trod path of assessment by an educational psychologist (who gave an excellent detailed and helpful report), and then extra tutoring for our son. Once again, we found this support invaluable. James's teacher was superb, and concentrated on phonology and a systematic approach to spelling.

However, in a moment of reflection one day it struck me, as I explained in my introduction, that within three generations of my own family those relatives who had been breast-fed the longest were less likely to display symptoms of dyslexia and other learning disorders. Some family members had not been breast-fed at all; one had been breast-fed for as long as two and a half years. (And it is important to note that even prolonged breast-feeding did not completely protect from the genetic predisposition to developing dyslexia.)

One of the notable features of breast milk is that it provides the long-chain polyunsaturated fatty acids—the LCPs—ready-formed, as well as the shorter-chain, precursor essential fatty acids, the EFAs. So I began to wonder if dyslexia could be due to a deficiency of LCPs in early life. I asked myself if children with dyslexia could be deficient in LCPs because of the diets of their mothers during pregnancy. And why would that be? Could it be that dyslexics cannot make enough of the LCPs from the precursor EFAs? Could such a deficiency interfere with the sensory input needed to read and write? So many questions needed answers.

## THE FIRST STUDY

To investigate the proposition that a mother's diet during pregnancy influences whether her child develops dyslexia, I enlisted the aid of my undergraduate students. Over a two-year period we looked at two groups of mothers with sons between ages eight and ten. One group's boys had been diagnosed with dyslexia; the other group comprised the mothers of their nondyslexic classmates. The mothers—more than one hundred of them—were given a comprehensive questionnaire containing questions related to specific fats.

The goal was to assess whether, during their pregnancies, the mothers of the dyslexic children had eaten foods with a lower supply of certain fatty acids. We developed, therefore, a scoring system to estimate the amounts of essential fatty acids and LCPs they had consumed. We were particularly interested in the ratio of omega-3 to omega-6 fatty acids.

The result was that the mothers of the dyslexic children were significantly more likely to have had a diet low in omega-3 fatty acids. The study also showed that in the women who had a family history of dyslexia, their diet had not made any difference. In these cases, it didn't matter if they had been eating foods rich in EFAs. This was an important finding. It supported my working hypothesis that the women with such a predisposition were obviously getting the precursor fatty acids in their diet but were not able to convert them to DHA and AA, the longer-chain form demanded by the hungry brain.

Of course, the study was based on the mothers' recollection of what their diet had been while pregnant approximately ten years earlier. It can be argued, therefore, that the data was not completely reliable, although I'm personally convinced that most mothers would clearly remember their dietary habits at such a meaningful time in their lives. In my view, they would definitely be able to accurately recollect if they had regularly eaten fish, the type of fish they had consumed, whether they had used butter instead of margarine, the brand of margarine they had used, and the type of vegetable oil they had preferred for cooking. Interestingly, although the mothers initially expressed some doubt over whether they would be able to remember their dietary habits, when they saw the actual questions they did not find answering them too difficult. Regardless, the outcome of the study was sufficient to suggest that there might indeed be a link between certain fatty acids and dyslexia, and that further research was warranted.

## SEEING THE LIGHT

Having shown that the mothers of dyslexic children, while pregnant, had eaten a diet low in omega-3 fatty acids, my next step was to look for evidence of long-chain fatty acid deficiency in dyslexics themselves. I wanted a biological measure for deficiency, a test that could not only quickly demonstrate whether there was a deficit, but also whether subsequent supplementation with certain fatty acids helped dyslexic individuals. I knew that the long-chain polyunsaturated fatty acid DHA is extremely important for vision. In fact, the retina has the highest percentage of DHA of any organ in the body. Its rod cells contain a stack of disks of phospholipid membrane and DHA makes up 60 percent of its fatty acid composition. All of these disks are replaced every ten to thirty days, which creates a huge demand for a continuing supply of DHA. Even though the retina is very efficient at conserving DHA, if any tissue would be likely to suffer from DHA deficiency, I knew it would be the retina.

The rod cells of the retina enable us to see in dim light—that is, night vision. (They are also important for peripheral vision and movement detection.) It seemed, therefore, that the best way to assess whether dyslexics had a DHA deficiency was to measure how their vision adapted to the dark. As a result, we took twenty young adults—male and female—between ages eighteen and twenty-six. Ten were dyslexic; ten were not. One of their eyes was covered, then bright light was shone into the other eye to bleach the retina, and the room was darkened. Using a piece of equipment called the Friedmann Visual Field Analyzer, at one-minute intervals we monitored whether they could see very brief flashes of light of varying intensity (measured as density units). At first they could see only the brightest flashes, but gradually, over a period of twenty minutes, they could see much dimmer light flashes. Their eyes had adapted to light of low intensity. Measurements were continued until no further adaptation was observed. Because dark adaptation can be influenced by a number of nutrients (especially vitamin A and zinc), the subjects were asked to keep a food diary and the intake of these nutrients was estimated. There was no difference in diet between the two groups. Throughout the test, at every time point, the dyslexics displayed significant and surprisingly poorer ability to adapt to the dark than the controls. (The poor adaptation to dark, by the way, could explain why children with dyslexia often say they are afraid of the dark; they cannot see as well as other children can.)

So, could this difficulty in adjusting to the dark be because dyslexics are deficient in DHA? What would happen if they were given DHA?

## FOUR OUT OF FIVE AND ONE OUT OF FIVE

For the next piece of the puzzle to fall into place we needed to supplement dyslexics with DHA to see if there would be any positive impact. Therefore, for one month, five dyslexics and five non-

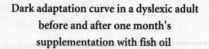

Dark adaptation curve in a dyslexic adult
before and after one month's
supplementation with fish oil

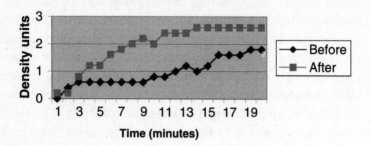

Time (minutes)

dyslexic controls were each given fish oil capsules containing a total of 480 milligrams of DHA per day and only traces of vitamins A and D. Their ability to adapt to the dark was then reexamined. Quite dramatically, four out of five dyslexic subjects supplemented with DHA displayed consistent and significant improvement in their ability to adjust to the dark. In fact, they were able to accommodate dimmer light equally as well as the nondyslexics. The one dyslexic who did not respond was an interesting case. She did not have poor dark adaptation at the outset, but we discovered that she habitually consumed large amounts of mackerel, so her diet was already rich in DHA.

Fish oil DHA supplementation had no benefit whatsoever for four of the nondyslexic control subjects, but the fifth nondyslexic subject did improve. It turned out that he was a fairly strict vegetarian whose normal diet was low in DHA. The discovery that he also improved was totally unexpected, because we did not know that he was a vegetarian, and this, therefore, added even further weight to the positive outcome of supplementation.

The rod cells of the retina are not only important for dark adaptation, they are also the photoreceptors of the magnocellular (large cell) pathway, the visual system that processes rapid stimuli (much faster than the blink of an eye). Using functional magnetic resonance imaging (fMRI), Professor John Stein at Oxford University has provided evidence that this system is impaired in dyslexia. There is no concrete proof, as yet, that improving the function of the photoreceptors (125 million in the retina of each eye) through DHA supplementation will also improve central processing deficits. But this is a likely outcome since synapse membranes, the junctions between nerve cells, contain high concentrations of DHA that need to be replenished.

## THE DYSPRAXIA DISCOVERY

After the medical publication *The Lancet* published my findings with the dyslexia group, the story was picked up by major British newspapers and the Reuters news agency. It then found its way into publications across the world and I was bombarded with letters from a dozen different countries. Out of the blue, a parent in the United Kingdom contacted me to ask if supplementation with long-chain polyunsaturated fatty acids would help his dyspraxic child. When he tried it, and the child responded favorably, members of the Dyspraxia Foundation in Bournemouth, England, wanted to test the supplement with a whole group of children.

From a scientific standpoint my preference was to conduct a double-blind, placebo-controlled trial so that none of us would know whether a particular child was receiving an active supplement or just a dummy capsule. However, despite all my persuasive powers, the parents declined to participate in a trial where some of the children did not get the real thing. Unfortunate, but understandable.

In the subsequent study, a total of fifteen dyspraxic children, eleven boys and four girls between the ages of five and twelve, received a mixture of omega-3 and omega-6 LCPs over a four-month period. The supplement provided a daily total of 480 milligrams of DHA, 35 milligrams of arachidonic acid, 96 milligrams gamma linolenic acid, 80 milligrams vitamin E, and 24 milligrams of thyme oil. Before and after supplementation, the children's motor skills were examined with the ABC Movement Assessment Battery for Children, a test that is regularly used to evaluate treatment interventions by physiotherapists and occupational therapists. The test is just as appropriate for measuring the result of nutritional supplementation. In addition, because of the overlap between dyspraxia and ADHD, the children's behavior was assessed by their parents using the Conners' Parent Rating Scales.

The ABC test has two parts. One part consists of a checklist that is completed by an adult familiar with the child (in this instance, a parent). The second part consists of a series of objective measures assessing manual dexterity, ball skills, and balance and is completed by the therapist. At the outset, the checklist scores for all of the children indicated a marked degree of movement difficulty. A similar degree of difficulty was found with the objective measures.

We had the children perform an assortment of tests. We assessed manual dexterity, for instance, by having them draw a line through a maze or around a flower trail, trying to keep within the parallel lines. We tested balance by having them stand on one leg or jump into squares—a little bit like hopscotch—with instructions not to land on the lines. We had them walk heel to toe. We counted the number of times they could catch a ball or successfully throw beanbags into a box on the ground. We had children screw nuts onto bolts and timed them in the process. There were also some pegboard tests. The kinds of tests, and their degree of difficulty, depended upon the age of the child.

After four months of LCP supplementation the children were reexamined using the same battery of tests. Overall, there were

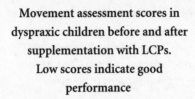

Movement assessment scores in
dyspraxic children before and after
supplementation with LCPs.
Low scores indicate good
performance

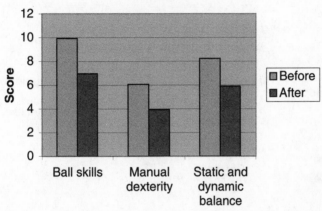

statistically significant improvements in all areas of measurement. Only one child failed to improve on the original checklist score and three did not change much on the objective measures. The children's behavior, as measured by the Conners' Parent Rating Scales, also improved and they were significantly less anxious.

The improvements in ball skills, manual dexterity, and balance, as well as the parent's checklist score, were very encouraging. You would be right, of course, to argue that the parents were wanting—and maybe expecting—to see such improvements. However, the manner in which the study was conducted, whereby the parents completed the second checklist without reference to the first, provides reasonable assurance that they were independently assessing their child's performance four months apart. I think it is fair to say that few people would remember

Average ABC total impairment scores and
checklist scores in dyspraxic children
before and after four months'
supplementation with LCPs. Low scores
indicate good performance

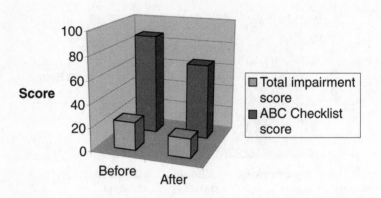

where they checked a box four months previously. Each record of the objective measures, such as how many balls they caught out of ten throws, or how long they took to complete a pegboard test, was subsequently transformed into a score. These records, too, were scored without knowledge of whether they referred to the first or second test. Overall, the total impairment score, which is the sum of scores for ball skills, manual dexterity, and static and dynamic balance, also improved as shown in the figure on page 111.

I was not too surprised when all of the results were collected because, in the meantime, a pharmacist had phoned me to tell of the quick and dramatic improvements in his eight-year-old son. After just the initial week of supplementation, the little boy had become calmer and his balance was better. After several more weeks he could catch a ball that was thrown at him and hit a ball with a baseball bat. He could also carry liquid in an uncovered cup without spilling the contents, a skill he had not previously acquired despite his years. His teacher, unaware that he was on LCP supplementation, reported that he was less disruptive in class. And he was actually volunteering to read to his mother, a very unusual occurrence in a child with a learning disorder.

For the children in the study there were other benefits, too. One little boy's frequent and severe temper tantrums became a thing of the past. Young Ben Cahill's uncontrollable tantrums had had a devastating effect on his family, his mother, Margaret, told me. Six-year-old Ben had always been extremely inflexible and disruptive. His routine could not be changed. He would flatly refuse to change places at the dinner table to accommodate a guest, and on one memorable occasion overnight visitors had left early because of his behavior. During the second month of the study, Margaret took Ben and some friends to the zoo. When she got there she realized she did not have much money with her and warned the children that they would not be able to have ice cream later. It was a hot, sticky summer's day and by the end of the day the children were naturally clamoring for ice cream. Hesitantly, Ben's mother reminded them that she had said there could be no ice cream, and waited for the inevitable outburst from Ben. Instead, he just shrugged his little shoulders and said, "Oh, dear. Silly me. I forgot." No tantrum. And that was the point at which she knew that LCP supplementation was really working. "Words failed me," recalled Margaret. "My friend and I stared at each other in amazement." Ben has continued to improve. "His behavior has transformed. Now he's such fun to have around," says his relieved mother.

Another child, severely constipated throughout her young life, found that that problem resolved itself with supplementation. Conversely, two others who had frequently soiled their pants at an age when they should have long outgrown this problem found that this was no longer an issue. It was fascinating to note that these other benefits could be attributed to the fact that motor skills are related to ways in which nerves control the muscles. Imagine what a meaningful difference this made to the lives of these children and their parents. Imagine the joy expressed to me by the parents of these children. Not all of the children responded to the same degree, but for some the improvements were so dramatic that when they returned for occupational therapy they no longer met the criteria that made them eligible for treatment by the British National Health Service. That gives you a measure of the progress they had made in just four months of supplementation.

## ATTENDING TO ADHD

At the same time as I was conducting my work with dyslexics and dyspraxics, researchers in the United States were exploring the importance of essential fatty acids in children with ADHD. Intriguingly, this all stemmed from the observations of British great-grandmother Vicki Colquhoun and her daughter, Sally Bunday. Although Colquhoun and Bunday had no scientific or medical qualifications, they did have a strong personal interest in ADHD and had founded the UK-based Hyperactive Children's Support Group. The results of a survey they had initiated in West Sussex, England, led them to develop the idea that ADHD might be the result of a deficiency of LCPs.

Their observations were drawn from reports that most of a large group of hyperactive children were thirstier than non-ADHD kids, urinated more frequently, and had dry skin and hair. The children also had histories of other conditions that were known to be relieved by LCP supplementation, such as asthma, eczema, and other allergies. Colquhoun and Bunday could not find any evidence of a dietary deficiency in the parents' intake of EFAs and proposed that there might be a problem in the conversion of EFAs to LCPs. They argued their proposition so persuasively that they managed to get it published in a 1981 edition of the scientific publication *Medical Hypotheses.*

The first clinical evidence substantiating their theory that ADHD children had low levels of DHA and AA did not come for another six years, until the work of Dr. E. A. Mitchell and colleagues was published in *Clinical Pediatrics.* This group compared forty-eight hyperactive children with forty-nine controls matched on an age and sex basis. They found that the hyperactive children had significantly lower levels of the LCPs docosahexaenoic acid (DHA), dihomogammalinolenic acid (DGLA), and arachidonic acid (AA) in their blood cell membranes. Calling for further research, Mitchell and colleagues said that their findings had possible therapeutic and diagnostic implications.

Another eight years would go by, however, before a group at Purdue University decided to seek further clinical substantiation. The Purdue studies were inspired by the interest of Laura Stevens, who selected the subject as part of her master's degree. Fortunately, she says, Dr. John Burgess joined the faculty at the same time as she was pursuing her degree and took the project on. Initially, these researchers compared fifty-three ADHD boys with forty-three non-ADHD youngsters, all between the ages of six and twelve. Their work, published in the *American Journal of Clinical Nutrition* in 1995, showed that the ADHD children:

- displayed clinical signs of LCP deficiency such as excessive thirst and the need to urinate frequently, and
- had much lower levels of AA and DHA in their red blood cell membranes even though, like the control group, they consumed plenty of the LA and ALA precursors in their diet. It looked like they were less able to convert LA and ALA into the long-chain derivatives AA and DHA. They also had more omega-6 DPA in the membranes. This is classically found when an individual is deficient in DHA.

Omega-3 long-chain polyunsaturated fatty acids in red blood cell
membranes of boys with ADHD compared with boys without ADHD

### Docosahexaenoic acid (DHA)

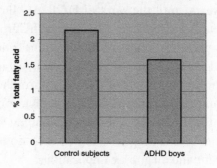

### Omega-3 docosapentaenoic
### acid (Omega-3 DPA)

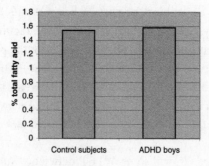

**Omega-6 long-chain polyunsaturated fatty acids in red blood cell membranes of boys with ADHD compared with boys without ADHD**

### Adrenic acid (AdrA)

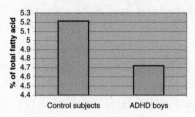

### Omega-6 docoasapentaenoic acid (Omega-6 DPA)

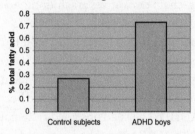

### Arachidonic acid (AA)

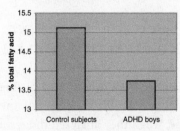

The ADHD boys were also:

- less likely to have been breast-fed (or had been breast-fed for shorter lengths of time) and
- more likely to suffer from asthma and other health problems

These findings with ADHD were completely consistent with my own results with dyslexics and dyspraxics. Examination of the fatty acid composition of the diets of these children indicated that there was not just a simple dietary deficiency of essential fatty acids, which could explain the results. It appears that children with ADHD are less able to convert the precursor essential fatty acids linoleic acid (LA) and alpha-linolenic acid (ALA) from their food, to the long-chain derivatives arachidonic acid (AA), adrenic acid (AdrA), and docosahexaenoic acid (DHA).

When I read the Purdue findings I could hardly believe my eyes. They had shown that the boys with ADHD were less likely to have been breast-fed. If they had been breast-fed it had been for a shorter duration. And the longer the child had been breast-fed the less severe the ADHD. They had observed systematically in a large group of boys with ADHD what I had observed in my own family, the touchstone of my research.

## BEHAVIOR, LEARNING, AND HEALTH PROBLEMS

The Purdue researchers then went on to further investigate the behavior, learning, and health problems of the boys they had studied. This time, when they analyzed the results, they divided the group of one hundred six- to twelve-year-old boys into those with high and low levels of omega-3 fatty acids in the blood. This was instead of comparing boys with ADHD and controls without

ADHD. The researchers asked parents and teachers to rate the children on the Conners' Parent and Teacher Rating Scales, the most commonly used behavior assessment tool for childhood behavior problems.

Published in the medical journal *Physiology and Behavior* in 1996, the study showed that the boys with lower levels of omega-3 fatty acids reported a significantly greater frequency of symptoms associated with LCP deficiencies including increased thirst, frequent urination, and dry skin. They also displayed significantly greater behavioral problems with more frequent and excessive temper tantrums. And they had greater difficulty falling asleep and getting up in the morning. Parents rated the LCP-deficient children as having significantly greater learning problems, and teachers noted overall lower academic ability and poorer math ability. Commented the research team: "These results, together with other previous descriptive studies, support a relationship between omega-3 fatty acid status and behavior in children that parallels what has been reported with rats and monkeys." Meanwhile, other researchers were beginning to investigate various aspects of fatty acid status and its connection to behavior.

## THE JAPANESE CONNECTION

Japanese researchers, for instance, validated a connection between fatty acid consumption and behavior by studying a normal group of people who had no significant health or learning problems. In a placebo-controlled, double-blind trial at the Toyama Medical and Pharmaceutical University, they gave forty-one male and female students fish oil capsules containing either 1.5 to 1.8 grams of DHA a day for three months or placebo capsules with very little DHA.

The study was arranged to end during the students' final

exams, a time when they would be expected to be going through acute mental stress. The group of students who did not receive the high DHA supplement exhibited significant extra aggression against others. The group supplemented with DHA was no more aggressive than when they had started the trial. Another piece of the puzzle had fallen into place proving a connection between LCP supplementation and an improvement in behavior. Fascinatingly, this research group went on to investigate if fish oil supplements prevented aggression under nonstressful conditions. They found that the supplements did not help in such conditions. Now we also knew that supplements were particularly helpful in stressed individuals.

So the picture was becoming a little clearer. Let's recap what we have learned so far.

1. I had discovered that mothers of dyslexic children had, while pregnant, been on a diet low in omega-3 fatty acids compared to the mothers of nondyslexics.

2. I had found that a group of young adult dyslexics had poor night vision and were probably deficient in DHA.

3. When dyslexics were given 480 milligrams of DHA a day as fish oil—for just a month—their ability to see in the dark became the same as that of nondyslexics.

4. Dyspraxic children, after four months of daily supplementation with 480 milligrams DHA from fish oil together with evening primrose oil, showed significant improvements in a whole battery of tests as well as behavior.

5. In a study comparing hyperactive children with controls, the hyperactive kids had significantly lower levels of LCPs in their red blood cell membranes.

6. The first Purdue study found that ADHD boys had clinical signs of LCP deficiency and lower levels of AA and DHA in their red blood cell membranes than non-ADHD boys

did. The ADHD boys were also less likely to have been breast-fed and more likely to suffer from asthma and other health problems.

7. The second Purdue study demonstrated that boys with lower levels of omega-3 fatty acids had significantly greater frequency of symptoms associated with LCP deficiency and displayed greater behavioral problems.

8. And, finally, two Japanese studies showed fatty acid supplementation helped people's behavior in stressful rather than non-stressful conditions.

Study by study, piece by piece, intriguing evidence was establishing an interconnected pattern. What would happen next?

## A CONTRARY RESULT

The next published research, prompted by the Purdue studies, also looked into the relationship between LCP status and ADHD. This study—a collaboration between the Mayo Clinic in Rochester, Minnesota, and Baylor College of Medicine in Houston, Texas—has been very helpful in narrowing down the specific "formula" that will help alleviate this disorder. In the study, forty-six children ages six to twelve completed the trial, split evenly between those who were given a DHA supplement of 345 milligrams a day for four months and those who received a placebo. All of the children had previously been on stimulant medication.

Researchers, led by Dr. Robert Voigt, reported that the DHA levels in the blood of children receiving DHA supplementation rose by 300 percent, but, unlike the Purdue subjects, there did not appear to be any improvement in their ADHD symptoms. Why not? This may be because the children were only supplemented with DHA, the source of which was micro algae, not fish oil. This means that the supplement used in this trial would not have contained any other LCPs, such as eicosapentaenoic acid (EPA) and arachidonic acid (AA), which are found in fish oil supplements. The supplement used would also not have contained any of the gammalinolenic acid (GLA) provided by the evening primrose oil. As we are not completely certain which LCPs are important and in what amounts, these other LCPs, in addition to DHA, may have an important function.

While this kind of research in the United States has focused on ADHD, U.K. researchers have primarily been looking at the connection with dyslexia.

## PEERING INSIDE THE DYSLEXIC BRAIN

Scientists asked themselves how else could the link between long-chain polyunsaturated fatty acid deficiency and dyslexia be validated? Into the jigsaw puzzle stepped a team at Oxford University, led by senior research fellow and honorary lecturer in psychology Dr. Alexandra Richardson and, from London's Hammersmith Hospital, senior lecturer and consultant in psychiatry Dr. Basant Puri and his colleagues.

Analyzing blood samples, as performed in earlier studies, allows researchers to measure the fatty acid composition of cell membranes, but it cannot tell what is happening inside the brain itself. So Richardson and Puri elected to peer inside the brains of living subjects—using phosphorus 31 functional magnetic resonance spectroscopy (MRS), a powerful and safe brain imaging technique—and watch the chemical processes "at work." It was the first-ever use of this technique for dyslexia research.

Richardson and Puri specifically set out to test the hypothesis that "membrane phospholipid metabolism" is abnormal in dyslexia. As I explained earlier, phospholipids are important fatty substances that form the structure of nerve membranes. In their trial with twelve dyslexics and ten nondyslexic controls, these researchers found altered brain chemistry in the dyslexics—an increase in a chemical called phosphomonoesters, which appears to indicate a reduced incorporation of fatty acids into phospholipid membranes. Their conclusion: "The metabolism of membrane phospholipids is heavily influenced by their EFA composition; so the present findings are also consistent with EFA deficiency in dyslexia, for which there is already some evidence. The importance of the long-chain polyunsaturated fatty acids such as DHA for visual and cognitive development is increasingly being recognized. It would, therefore, not be altogether surprising if they were to play some role in a range of neurodevelopmental disorders, including dyslexia."*

## THE SWEDISH CONTRIBUTION

Meanwhile, in Sweden, yet another piece of the puzzle was coming together, not only giving us evidence of the beneficial effects of supplementation but also indicating the time frame for results to be experienced. In 1998, researchers Lars Lindmark and Turid Styrsven conducted a five-month study with nineteen children, sixteen of whom were dyslexic; five were recognized as having slow physical development. In fourteen children there was a family history of learning disorders. All of the children, who were between the ages of nine and seventeen, were given a mixture of fish oil and evening primrose oil providing 480 milligrams of DHA a day. They found increased reading speed following such LCP supplementation.

Of great interest, however, is the time frame in which parents

*In this quotation, the authors are using the term "EFA" to include LCPs.

reported positive results. After the first six weeks, five out of the nineteen (26 percent) had already seen a difference. After twelve weeks, the number was up to twelve (63 percent). After sixteen weeks, thirteen of the children (76 percent) had responded positively, and at the end of the trial—twenty weeks—seventeen out of the nineteen (89 percent) had benefited from supplementation. This really proves the point that instant results cannot be expected. Varying lengths of time are required for the LCP content of body tissues to be raised to sufficient levels to make a difference.

## ONGOING RESEARCH

The most recent ADHD research has been carried out at Purdue University and the most recent dyslexic research at Oxford University. In the Purdue study, which is awaiting publication in a scientific journal, fifty children displaying symptoms of LCP deficiency were randomized blindly to one of two groups. One group received an LCP supplement, the second group received a placebo.

Parents' assessment of their child's behavior and frequency of LCP deficiency symptoms were obtained at the beginning and at two, four, eight, twelve, and sixteen weeks. Objective behavioral assessments and tests of cognitive ability were conducted at the beginning and end of the study. Teachers' assessments of both behavior and scholastic performance were obtained prior to the start of the study and after about two months of supplementation. Preliminary results from this trial were presented by Dr. John Burgess at a National Institutes of Health conference in Washington, D.C., in 1998. The results were encouraging. Some groups of ADHD boys who had received a high DHA fish oil and evening primrose oil supplement showed improvement in behavior, but not across all measures.

Commenting on the trial, one expert familiar with the results,

Dr. L. Eugene Arnold of Ohio State University, was cautiously positive about the benefits of LCP supplementation and suggested that the research to date merited further controlled trials. At the same time, Dr. Arnold, who conducted a major review of many alternative approaches to treating ADHD, dismissed the results of other nutritional strategies such as simple elimination of sugar or candy from the diet, supplementation with amino acids, and megavitamin cocktails.

In a paper presented to an NIH conference, he reported that the Purdue trial "showed a trend of advantage for the supplement despite a huge placebo effect." Changes in serum phospholipid omega-3 acids correlated negatively with changes in Conner scores, he said. In other words, the less LCP in the blood, the worse the child's behavior.

Dr. Richardson and her team at Oxford University are collaborating on three large double-blind, placebo-controlled trials with a total of more than two hundred participants. One study consists of one hundred adults. Some have dyslexia; others are nondyslexic controls. The second study comprises a similarly large group of children, all with dyslexia. The third study, which has been completed, examined the value of LCP supplements in children attending a special school for children with specific learning disorders.

While the results of the first two studies are not yet available, some of the analysis of the baseline data has been conducted. This shows that the dyslexic adults displayed greater signs of long-chain fatty acid deficiency compared with the nondyslexics. In the group of dyslexic children, those that were more deficient in LCPs were found to be more behind in their reading. The reading lag was as much as thirty months in the highly deficient group.

In these first two trials, one group is receiving LCP supplementation and the other a placebo (dummy capsule) for six months. The placebo group will then switch to LCPs for six months while

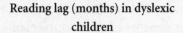

Reading lag (months) in dyslexic
children

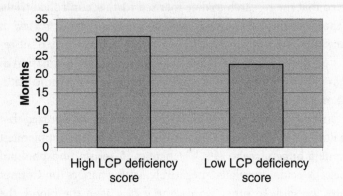

those already taking LCPs will continue with them for six months more. The subjects will be followed up with various tests at three-month intervals, so it can be assessed whether or not supplementation has been beneficial.

In the six-month-long school study, which has been completed, the children were divided into two groups. One group received supplementation for the initial three months while the other group received a placebo. For the next three months, the first group continued to receive LCP supplements and the second group was switched from the placebo to LCP supplements. This study design is called a single crossover study because only the placebo group changes its treatment halfway through. It is the only suitable design for observing the effect of LCPs since their effect continues for some weeks, if not months, after one stops taking them. During the period after supplementation, the individuals would still be affected by the previous supplementation because it takes time to deplete the body of LCPs and the results would not be clear-cut.

It is important to note that these three trials are all "double blind," which means that neither the observer nor the participant knows whether the participant is on the supplement or the placebo. This kind of study provides the ultimate proof of whether something is effective. And the answer for the use of LCPs in helping learning disorders is yes.

The results from the school study show that ADHD ratings are high in children with dyslexia and that signs of fatty acid deficiency are associated with both of the major types of ADHD: inattention and hyperactivity/impulsivity. The results of supplementation with LCPs are fascinating. At the beginning of this study there was no difference in the Conners' Parent Rating Scales between the placebo group and the LCP group. After twelve weeks, however, the LCP group displayed improvements in the average scores for cognitive problems, behavior problems, and anxiety. The children receiving the placebo showed no improvement.

When the placebo group was switched to LCPs they, too, displayed significant improvements while the children who had used LCPs continuously maintained their reduction of symptoms. All of these children were attending a school where the staff is skilled at helping children with specific learning difficulties. Nevertheless, improvements were only noted following LCP supplementation.

## WHERE DO WE GO FROM HERE?

Obviously, the most important question for individuals with ADHD, dyslexia, or dyspraxia is: Do LCP supplements work? We now know that they do. This question has been resolved by Dr. Richardson's major trial. The next important question is: Which supplements work best? We don't know for sure, but we do know that a combination of high DHA fish oil together with evening primrose oil is effective in relieving many of the features of these conditions.

The scientists, of course, want to know the cause of the problem. What is its biochemical mechanism? Is it that the desaturation and elongation of EFAs is defective, as seems to be the case? Or is it that the incorporation of LCPs into membrane phospholipids is at fault? Or maybe is it because membranes are being built and destroyed at a faster rate than normal, which creates a greater need for LCPs than can easily be met? Think of it in the same sort of way that a fast-burning fire needs more logs. We know there's a membrane difference because of the work of Richardson and the phosphorus 31 brain scan studies. Her group is now looking to see if they can change that membrane problem with supplementation. What a discovery that would be. It will be even more exciting if it is shown that supplementation changes areas of the brain that are used to process language. But that is all speculation until the experiments are conducted.

Will fatty acid supplementation work for everyone? No. Behavior problems, dyslexia, and dyspraxia can also be caused by brain injury from trauma or lack of oxygen. In these cases it is extremely unlikely that LCP supplementation will help. The Richardson studies have begun to show who benefits the most. The research does appear to show that just as many ADHD children and adults derive benefit from LCP supplementation (75 to 80 percent) as do from using a drug such as Ritalin. It is also clear that some aspects of these conditions respond more to supplementation than others.

I was especially interested to see that the results of the school study showed that anxiety was reduced following supplementation because that benefit was also evident in my own study with dyspraxic children. One might think that all of the children attending a school with teachers who understand their condition would have reduced anxiety. But the children only improved in this way when they were supplemented.

The supplements we are using now are a blunt tool. But they are effective for many. We have made more than the first step, but there is much more research needed in the whole area of the role of long-chain polyunsaturated fatty acids in early infant development, in childhood, and in adult life.

Now that I have covered the research substantiating the need for LCP supplementation, it's time to show how it can be put into practice.

# THE PLAN

THE PLAN

# CHAPTER 7

# SUPPLEMENTS— THE SIMPLE ANSWER

*DHA is part of what we might call: an Old diet for A New Millennium . . . restoring part of our ancestral diet is as easy as D-H-A!*

—JAMES J. GORMLEY, *DHA, A GOOD FAT: ESSENTIAL FOR LIFE*

It's actually as easy as LCP! As you've discovered, the single most effective and natural way to alleviate the symptoms of ADHD, dyslexia, and dyspraxia is to make sure you and your children are getting enough long-chain polyunsaturated fatty acids (LCPs) in your diet, especially DHA. This simple approach will make all the difference in the world. Consuming more of these "good" fats will win the battle for your child's mind, beating out the competing fats that "scramble" the brain. The LCPs will help to repair the faulty brain circuitry that impacts children with these learning disorders. But exactly how do you get enough of them?

As I revealed in Chapter 5, the natural food sources rich in LCPs are fish—salmon, mackerel, tuna, trout, sardines, and blue-fish. They provide a good supply of DHA and EPA, and small amounts of AA. But to obtain the amounts that are needed to combat learning disorders would mean frequent consumption of large quantities of such fish. Regularly eating any kind of fish would be a sensible and healthy part of anyone's normal diet. But some people find the cost to be prohibitive (especially if they want to eat salmon) and most, especially youngsters, just don't want to do so. Imagine trying to impose a diet of "fish, fish, and more fish" on a young child: "No, Johnny. You can't have a Big Mac. Have a nice big piece of mackerel, instead." It doesn't work. Also, in some places, it's not easy to buy this kind of fish.

In the following chapter I will, nevertheless, discuss sensible eating issues, pointing out foods that contain useful amounts of omega-3 LCPs, and also foods that contain unhelpful trans fatty acids. Adopting a healthy diet would be a valuable contribution to a healthy lifestyle. But we need to be realistic. For most people, taking LCP supplements is an ideal, easy, and cost-effective method of obtaining the same nutritional benefits. In any case, virtually all of the results reported in this book are based on studies in which patients consumed supplements rather than fish.

Still, I would be remiss not to point out that some nutritionists refuse to recommend supplementation—even when needs for specific nutrients are particularly high and it is hard to obtain them from food. Frankly, I find this to be a strange attitude. It's as though these nutritionists think they have somehow failed if they cannot put together menus of "real" food to achieve a particular nutritional goal. It is even more surprising when supplementing "at risk" groups and/or providing them with nutrient-enriched food has been responsible for successfully resolving so many health problems. One good example is the use of vitamin D supplements to help prevent rickets (which used to be called the "English disease"). Other examples are the addition of iodine to salt to forestall both goiter and the serious mental retardation associated with iodine deficiency, and the recommendation that women preparing for pregnancy take folic acid supplements to guard against their babies developing conditions such as spina bifida and anencephaly.

## Getting Started

So what LCPs should be taken and how much? The best evidence from the clinical trials so far suggests that a substantial quantity of LCPs is needed to foster appreciable changes in those who suffer from ADHD, dyslexia, and dyspraxia. We can say with some assurance that fish oil providing 480 milligrams of DHA a day appears to be effective for both children and adults. This also provides other LCPs such as EPA and AA.

Usually, individuals prefer to split their daily intake into half in the morning and the other half in the evening, but this is probably not necessary. Children under five need half of this amount. Older children should take the same dosage as adults because their nutritional needs per pound of body weight are comparatively higher than those of adults. The developing child is growing nerve tissue, as well as muscles and bone, and the long-chain polyunsaturated fatty acids are the building blocks needed to support this growth.

These amounts of LCPs should be taken for the first three months. After this time, most users can move on to a maintenance level of half of the starting dose. But it is important to make a commitment of at least three months and to persevere. Undoubtedly, once you've started your child on the supplementation program, you're going to be anxiously awaiting results. Please don't expect to see instant success. Your child has probably been deprived of the LCPs to such an extent that it will take some time for sufficient stores in his body to be replenished. While it is true that some individuals do notice benefits within weeks, many have found that it can take twelve weeks or longer. It all depends upon the individual. As children are growing fast, they will sometimes burn the fatty acid supplements as energy rather than allowing them to proceed to the membranes where they are really needed. In a child who is seriously deficient in LCPs, it may well take as long as three months to build up the amounts needed in all of the body's tissues. Therefore, you won't be able to make a realistic evaluation of LCP supplementation if you haven't given it three months.

Once you've moved on to the maintenance level, what's next? Is your child (or yourself) going to need to keep taking LCP supplements forever? Frankly, I don't yet have the evidence to show how long people will need to continue supplementation. Some people who have stopped taking supplements do notice deterioration after a month or two, but it is possible that once children have gone through their pubertal growth spurt they may require less. In their adult years, their bodies may well be able to make enough. Those people who find that they do not enjoy the same benefits when they go on a maintenance dosage need to stick with fish oil providing 480 mg of DHA per day. This is something that needs to be monitored on an individual basis. Some people are able to decrease the amount they are taking; others are not. The simplest solution? At the very least, keep taking the maintenance dosage. The possibility of side effects is remote and greatly outweighed by the general benefits to overall health in addition to helping the learning disorder.

Says Jeannette Ewin, author of *The Fats We Need To Eat:* "Essential fatty acids and their biological derivatives are the most exciting health and medical story of the decade. Learning to improve the quality of the fats we eat, and to use food supplements wisely, will make our lives healthier and longer."

People of all ages, from young children to the very elderly, can benefit from LCP supplementation. In general, however, supplements should not be given to children under the age of three unless specifically directed by a doctor. Of course, LCPs have been added to the milk given to premature babies, but in these situations great care is always taken to make sure the supplements have the right amounts of fatty acids in the right form. One of the concerns about giving fish oil supplements to the very young is that some fish oils, particularly the liver oils, may contain excessive amounts of the fat-soluble vitamins A and D. Taken in excess, vitamins A and D can be toxic and should, therefore, be avoided. The chance of reaching an excess level is much increased if children are given several multivitamin supplements that contain vitamins A and D, in addition to fish liver oils. To some extent, however, this is a nonissue, as most learning disorders are not identified this early, and the subject of LCP supplementation does not arise—though it is something of which you should be aware.

At the other end of the age scale I have an excellent illustration of how it's never too late to enjoy improvements from LCP supplementation. It came in a really heartwarming letter from the wife of a dyslexic gentleman in his seventies. She reported that after supplementation, to her great relief, he had begun to drive more safely at night. Apparently, he no longer weaved from side to side on the road! He also dressed faster in the morning. This, of course, not only demonstrates the benefit of supplementation in aiding night vision, but also in the movement skills needed for putting on clothes.

## THE RITALIN QUESTION

Before looking at specific forms of supplementation, I want to address one of the questions I am most frequently asked. It concerns children with ADHD who have been prescribed Ritalin or a similar drug. Many parents want to know if it is safe to take LCPs along with Ritalin. First, let me say that *you must consult with your physician if your child is taking stimulant medication and you wish to try any kind of LCP supplementation.* In fact, before making dietary changes, it is always advisable for anyone taking any kind of medication to discuss it with his or her doctor.

It is not ethical for me as a nutritionist to give medical advice to individuals, but I can offer some general advice: It is not just safe to take essential fatty acids—it is essential! The body cannot make its own supply so we have to consume foods (or supplements) that provide them. Furthermore, there have been numerous carefully monitored clinical studies in which omega-6 and omega-3 EFA and LCP supplements have been safely given not only to adults but also to premature babies, infants, children, mothers-to-be, nursing mothers, and even cancer patients.

Now, as to the question of taking LCPs as well as Ritalin: Many individuals have taken LCPs in addition to Ritalin and other stimulant medications prescribed for ADHD without any problems. Ritalin, in the form usually dispensed, is a relatively short-acting drug that hits peak activity about two hours after it is taken. The effect then gradually wears off, so that after four hours or so another dose is needed. LCP supplements, on the other hand, are a mixture of nutrients and it may be weeks or even months before they change the composition of nerve membranes enough to change behavior.

So, after commencing LCP supplementation, how would anyone know if it is making a difference? Here's what needs to be done. Closely monitor the child's behavior, paying particular attention in two different scenarios. First, before introducing the LCPs, observe the difference between the child's behavior when Ritalin is at the height of its potency, and when it is wearing off. Quite a few children, for instance, experience the so-called rebound effect in the evening when they may become disruptive, and may have difficulty falling asleep. Or some parents give their child a drug holiday every weekend—and that's when he's overly active. If, after supplementing the child and allowing some weeks to pass, he becomes calmer when he would usually become hyper, it is likely that the LCP supplementation is working. The parents should consult with the doctor to consider reducing the dose of Ritalin.

Second, attention should be given to the time when Ritalin would usually be most effective (roughly two hours after it is taken). After some weeks of supplementation, it may be found that two hours after taking Ritalin the child gets *even worse* when he's normally on his best behavior—and that's a very good sign! I know that some parents have had this happen and felt that the supplement was having an adverse effect. Nothing could be further from the truth. Paradoxically, if the child becomes more excitable and hyper, it shows that the LCP supplementation is working. This is a clear indication that the LCPs have helped change the composition of cell membranes so that they are more normal. The Ritalin is now working in the child in the same way it does with non-ADHD individuals. It is now being allowed to act as the stimulant it is!

It is extremely important to be aware of this fact and for parents to consult with the doctor so that he can approve and supervise a reduction in medication. With the physician's guidance, it may well be possible to reduce the dosage of Ritalin step by step and, as the child's behavior improves and his ability to focus gets better and better, phase it out completely.

## Choosing Your Supplement

What is the best form of LCP supplementation? There is a confusing selection of fatty acid supplements in the marketplace. You will find people promoting the respective merits of flaxseed oil, cod liver oil, micro algae, and fish oil supplements. Let me clear up the confusion. All of these supplements are good for your child's general health (and your own). But some are likely to be better than others in alleviating the symptoms of ADHD, dyslexia, and dyspraxia. So let's go through them one by one.

FLAXSEED OIL    Many people are strong proponents of the health benefits of flaxseed oil, which contains ALA, a shorter-chain omega-3 EFA. Most people's bodies can convert ALA into the longer-chain fatty acids EPA and DHA, but the conversion is slow. In individuals who for genetic reasons have higher needs for LCPs, such as those with ADHD, dyslexia, and dyspraxia—or when the needs for growth are high, as in childhood, pregnancy, and lactation—it is unlikely that enough DHA would be produced from the ALA. Studies have shown that it can take up to ten times as much ALA from flaxseed oil to get the same benefits as EPA and DHA from fish oil. Flaxseed oil is also very unstable and needs to be kept refrigerated for safety reasons, which may be inconvenient.

COD LIVER OIL    Cod liver oil and some other fish oils do contain DHA, but not as much as is found in fish oils from other tissues of the fish. They also provide relatively more EPA than DHA. It is not clear yet whether this is a disadvantage or advantage. Most fish liver oils, however, are less suitable as they contain more vitamins A and D. Superficially, this may seem advantageous, but it's not. LCP supplementation is a long-term undertaking and there is a chance of consuming a harmful excess of these fat-soluble vitamins, particularly if foods fortified with vitamins A and D or other multivitamin supplements are taken.

MICRO ALGAE    Some manufacturers have developed products with micro algae as the source of the DHA. They point out that this is ideal for strict vegetarians who do not want to eat fish products and who are generally deficient in DHA because it is missing from most plant-based foods. While micro algae is a good source of DHA, it does not contain other longer-chain LCPs such as AA and EPA that are found in fish oil. In some countries some manufacturers are now also producing micro algae sources of AA; these have mostly been used for fortifying formula milk for babies.

From the evidence available at present, to protect against the development of learning disorders and to help children who already have such challenges, fish oil is preferred to micro algae.

FISH OIL    The supplement most widely used in clinical trials concerning learning disorders has been a fish oil–based capsule marketed under the name of Efalex. Each capsule contains 60 milligrams of DHA and 5.25 milligrams of AA (from the fish oil) along with evening primrose oil supplying 12 milligrams of GLA. The supplement also includes EPA, but the amount is not declared. In addition, vitamin E and thyme oil are contained in the product as research has shown that such antioxidants help protect fatty acids in the body and aid the incorporation of fatty acids into the membranes. Other manufacturers have developed their own fish oil supplements, many of which are listed at the end of this chapter. The manufacturer of Efalex won the right to make the claim "for the dietary management of fatty acid deficiency in ADHD." It also has the license for a patent for LCPs to be used in the treatment of dyslexia and dyspraxia.

One concern I have heard is that fish oil can be contaminated with toxic chemicals such as PCBs, dioxin, and mercury that cause neurological defects in the fetus. Responsible manufacturers are well aware of the potential problem of contaminants in any food, whether fish, fish oil, or even flaxseed oil. They set extremely tight specifications and they regularly test to ensure that their suppliers have met their specifications. In general, it is in fish *liver* oils where this potential exists rather than in the marine oils derived from other parts of the fish. But because this is the case, manufacturers carefully monitor production. Make sure, however, that you purchase products from reputable companies. Contact the manufacturer and ask about their quality assurance procedures so you can be confident their products are free of contaminants. Any reliable company will have the information readily at hand and will be pleased to respond to your inquiry.

Most manufacturers have produced LCP supplements in small, easy-to-swallow pills or softgel capsules, forms that are the most economical. Children, however, often resist taking pills of any kind, and in this instance, may well find the fishy taste of the liquid inside the capsules offensive. Product formulators are obviously well aware of this and do their best to mask the taste, but LCPs are also being incorporated into more "eater-friendly" foods such as yogurt-coated bars that are ideal for kids to take to school in a lunch box. Delivering the LCPs in this format not only helps cover the fishy taste but is also more palatable from a social standpoint. It doesn't seem as if the children are "taking medicine." (DHA from micro algae has also been added to eggs, shakes, and other foods.) The downside is that these products are more expensive than softgel capsules.

Another strategy, if you have a young child who finds it difficult to swallow capsules, is to cut them open and mix the oil content with food (such as breakfast cereal). Parents have found all sorts of ways to encourage their children. Some have mixed the oil with drinks; others have tried disguising the flavor by mixing it with jam and serving it on a spoon. Bribery also sometimes helps!

Before proceeding to identify leading supplements that contain LCPs and telling you where to obtain them, I'd like to answer some specific questions about supplementation that I've received during my lectures.

### Can you take too much EFA or LCP as supplements?

It would be hard to "overdose" on either the shorter-chain essential fatty acids or the LCPs. What the brain and other tissues don't need will be burned as energy. There are some communities in the world where people consume far more LCPs—through eating large amounts of fish and marine mammals—than would be true for someone following the instructions on the supplement bottle. These people do not appear to suffer any harmful consequences. Nevertheless, you should carefully monitor what other ingredients may be contained in different products. As I mentioned earlier, you would not wish to digest too much of vitamins A and D if you take fish liver oils. In a few very rare inherited conditions, individuals are unable to process LCPs efficiently and in these cases LCP supplementation should be closely monitored.

### Should children already taking LCP supplements stop taking them before being tested for levels of DHA?

This is not really necessary. The test will obviously reflect levels based on supplementation, but will still be a helpful guide as to the children's current status. However, the relationship between blood indicators of LCP status and the severity of ADHD, dyslexia, or dyspraxia is not yet precisely understood. New research in this area is in progress and should be published in the next couple of years.

### Is it harmful to take children off LCPs for a little while and then put them back on?

No. Just as it takes time to build up the LCP content of membranes it takes time for it to decrease again.

### Is there a possibility of a buildup in the liver from taking too much DHA?

I am not aware of any hazard to the liver by taking "too much" DHA. The amounts recommended as supplements are well within the amounts recommended by official bodies such as the World Health Organization.

### Does supplementation with LCPs help people with Down's syndrome?

I know that some parents have been giving their Down's

syndrome children LCP supplements, and there are anecdotal reports of significant benefits. However, I am not aware of any clinical research that would prove the effectiveness of LCPs in Down's syndrome patients. Dr. Tuomas Westermarck in Finland has done some fascinating research on the importance of giving plenty of antioxidants to people with Down's syndrome. It may well be useful to provide LCPs as well as antioxidants to maintain healthy brain membranes.

### Is there any connection between evening primrose oil and seizures?

One of the leading supplements used in clinical trials contains a small amount of evening primrose oil. Some parents have expressed concern about the potential for seizures based on unfortunate and inaccurate stories floating around the Internet. In my search of the scientific and medical literature I have not uncovered any evidence to support this suggestion. Evening primrose oil is 99 percent fat. Of that, 69 percent is linoleic acid, an omega-6 essential fatty acid; roughly 8 percent is GLA, an omega-6 fatty acid. GLA is a normal metabolite of LA in the body where it is converted to DGLA, and then AA. Mother's milk contains LA and DGLA, so it is extremely unlikely that these fatty acids are inherently unsafe! Both LA and GLA are also found in infant formulas. An 11-pound baby consuming about a quart of formula a day would be consuming just as much GLA as a child on Efalex, an LCP supplement that contains some evening primrose oil. There are also some saturated fatty acids and oleic acid in evening primrose oil, but these are also found in human milk, so once again are unlikely to cause problems.

Since the mid-1970s, large amounts of evening primrose oil have been consumed worldwide, and to my knowledge no negative effects have been reported to government agencies. In extensive clinical trials of evening primrose oil with thousands of patients, there was no excess of seizures in the treated groups. So, how did this story about evening primrose oil originate? I can only speculate that it was the result of a misinterpretation of a clinical trial with schizophrenic patients in which a few patients consuming evening primrose oil had seizures. However, these patients had previously experienced seizures and the drugs they were taking were known to precipitate epileptic attacks. It is likely, therefore, that even the attacks that did occur were totally unrelated to evening primrose oil. Clearly, anyone on medication or with a history of seizures should consult his or her doctor before taking LCP supplements.

*I've heard that vitamin E can be toxic in large quantities. Is this true?*

It is very difficult to take too much of a water-soluble vitamin—because the body readily excretes any excess. But it is more difficult to rid the body of an excess of a fat-soluble vitamin like A, D, and E. The dangers of excess A and D are well recognized, but very few adverse effects from too much vitamin E have been observed. The Council for Responsible Nutrition in Washington, D.C., has said that vitamin E can be consumed in daily amounts as high as 66 international units per pound of body weight. For a three-year-old child this is equivalent to about 3,000 IU per day. Concerned parents, knowing the weight of their child, can easily calculate whether there is an appropriate amount of vitamin E in a supplement.

Many manufacturers now give vitamin E content by weight rather than the old-fashioned international units. One IU of vitamin E is equivalent to 0.67 milligrams of tocopherol equivalents. (Tocopherol is the chemical name for vitamin E. The term "tocopherol equivalents" is used because there are eight tocopherol compounds that have slightly different chemical structures, but all have vitamin E activity in the body). So, 300 IU would be 201 milligrams of vitamin E.

### *Does supplementation with LCPs help people with obsessive compulsive disorder?*

I am not aware of any research with regard to LCP supplementation and OCD. However, I do know of one dyslexic who developed OCD acutely and severely at puberty. He was given the usual medication for OCD that influences the metabolism of serotonin, one of the neurotransmitters in the brain. He also took LCP supplements for dyslexia. Within three months he no longer required medication for OCD. His doctor commented that such a fast recovery was unusual and that the LCP supplements may well have been helpful. I have also heard a few anecdotal reports of improvement in Tourette's syndrome, a condition that frequently occurs in tandem with OCD. More research is needed to confirm or deny the possibility that LCPs help these conditions.

# PRODUCTS

You're ready to begin LCP supplementation, but where do you turn? The leading recommended brands of supplements are available in health food stores, pharmacies, and supermarkets throughout the country. In some instances, you can obtain them directly from the manufacturers, and, of course, there's the Internet. For your convenience, I have listed the products with which I am most familiar.

It is really quite difficult to compare products because manufacturers do not declare all of the nutrients provided by the ingredients listed on the package. The EPA content of many fish oil products is often not declared, even though it would be very surprising if EPA was not present. Others don't give values for vitamins A and D. Rarely is the LA content of evening primrose oil declared. I have tried to help by listing for each product the ingredients, the nutrition claims made, and the manufacturer's instructions for use. I have also provided contact details for the manufacturers so you can get in touch with them if you need more information.

## Efalex

A largely fish oil–based supplement, rich in DHA, Efalex is the product that was used in the clinical trials with dyslexia and dyspraxia. It was also the supplement in the Purdue University ADHD supplementation study. In some countries a lemon-lime liquid version of Efalex is available. This is particularly good for young children.

INGREDIENTS   high DHA fish oil, evening primrose oil, vitamin E, and thyme oil; capsule shell: gelatin and glycerin.

NUTRIENT CLAIMS   Each capsule contains 60 mg DHA (docosahexaenoic acid), 12 mg GLA (gamma-linolenic acid), 5.25 mg AA (arachidonic acid), 1 mg thyme oil, and 7.5 IU vitamin E.

MANUFACTURER'S INSTRUCTIONS   When taking the product for the first time it is recommended that children under the age of five have two to three capsules both morning and evening for a period of twelve weeks (or two teaspoons daily of the liquid). Children over five and adults should embark on a twelve-week course of four capsules in the morning and four in the evening (or two teaspoons of the liquid in the morning and the same at night). After twelve weeks, the recommended maintenance course for children under five is one to two capsules each morning and evening (or one teaspoon daily of the liquid). For children over five and adults, the dosage is two capsules each morning and evening (or two teaspoons daily of the liquid). The capsules or liquid should be consumed with food or drink.

If necessary, the capsules can be cut open and the contents mixed with food or drink. This formulation is free from sugar, yeast, milk derivatives, cornstarch, preservatives, and artificial colors and flavors.

## Efanatal

Specially formulated to provide fatty acids before, during, and after pregnancy, Efanatal is especially valuable during the last trimester of pregnancy, when fetal brain and nervous system growth are remarkably rapid.

**INGREDIENTS**    fish oil, evening primrose oil, vitamin E, gelatin, glycerol, carmine color, titanium dioxide color, ammonium phosphatide, ascorbyl palmitate (vitamin C).

**NUTRIENT CLAIMS**    Each capsule of Efanatal contains 53.5 mg DHA, 4.7 mg AA, 20 mg GLA, 7.51 IU vitamin E.

**MANUFACTURER'S INSTRUCTIONS**    The suggested daily intake is two capsules per day with food or drink.

Efamol Nutraceuticals, a company that was acquired by the Dutch-based international concern Nutricia, developed Efalex and Efanatal. The company defines the word "nutraceuticals" as pharmaceutical-grade nutritional products. This means, it says, that the products they produce are backed by rigorous scientific research and clinical studies.

AVAILABILITY   Efalex and Efanatal are available at RiteAid, GNC, Drugstore.com, and health food stores throughout the country.

MANUFACTURER
Nutricia USA
Clearwater, FL 33762
Phone: 877-458-6400
Web: www.efamol.com

# Neuromins®

A substantial number of clinical trials have been conducted using micro-algae, a vegetable source of DHA produced by Martek Biosciences. Most of the research has focused on investigating the DHA needs of newborns for brain and visual development, as well as mental and cardiovascular health in adult groups. Martek's products are marketed under the name Neuromins and each contains essentially the same ingredients, other than the amount of DHA. Capsules containing between 100 mg and 500 mg of DHA are presented in a sunflower-oil base with antioxidant protection supplied by vitamins C and E. Neuromins DHA capsules provide an organic vegetable source of DHA cultivated under strictly controlled conditions. They contain no artificial colors, preservatives, or EPA.

## NEUROMINS

INGREDIENTS   high oleic acid sunflower oil, docosahexaenoic acid from algal oil, ascorbyl palmitate (vitamin C), mixed natural tocopherol (vitamin E), mixed carotenoids, gelatin capsule shell.

**NUTRIENT CLAIMS**  500 mg capsules providing 100 mg of DHA and promoted as a "dietary supplement for the brain."

**MANUFACTURER'S INSTRUCTIONS**  Recommended dosage is one capsule a day as a nutritional supplement taken with a meal.

## NEUROMINS 200

**NUTRIENT CLAIMS**  500 mg capsules providing 200 mg of DHA.

**MANUFACTURER'S INSTRUCTIONS**  Recommended as a one-a-day "dietary supplement for the brain."

## NEUROMINSPL

NeurominsPL is essentially the same product as Neuromins 200 (containing 200 mg of DHA per capsule) except that it is promoted as a "dietary supplement of DHA for pregnant and lactating women." It is said to elevate levels of DHA in the blood supplying the placenta during pregnancy and in breast milk during lactation. This, in turn, elevates the baby's level of DHA. NeurominsPL also replenishes a woman's store of DHA, which is depleted by the developing infant during pregnancy.

## NEUROMINS FOR KIDS

**NUTRIENT CLAIMS**  Each 250 mg capsule provides 100 mg of DHA.

**MANUFACTURER'S INSTRUCTIONS**  One capsule a day for children. Each small, easy-to-swallow 250 mg capsule should be taken with a meal.

**AVAILABILITY**  Neuromins DHA products are available in health food stores under various brand names including Nature's Way, Solgar, Source Naturals, Solaray, Natrol, Tree of Life, Vitamin World, Whole Foods, BioDynamax, Vitamin Shoppe, and Your Life. The Natrol brand can also be found at Eckerd's, Osco, Sav-On, and Lucky, and there is a Safeway Select brand at Safeway. Also check out the Puritan's Pride and Vitamin Shoppe catalogs.

Neuromins 200 and Neuromins for Kids are available in health food stores from Source Naturals and by mail order. NeurominsPL is primarily available by mail order. Neuromins is also available under the name "Eye-Q" from distributors of a person-to-person sales company: Royal BodyCare, Inc., 2301 Crown Court, Irving, TX 75038-4305. Phone: 972-893-4000. Fax: 972-893-4111. www.royalbodycare.org

**MANUFACTURER**
Martek Biosciences Corporation
6480 Dobbin Road
Columbia, MD 21045
888-662-6339
Web: www.martekbio.com

## Learning Factors

This product is promoted as a "nutritional support for learning, attention, and concentration." Produced by the Canadian company Natural Factors (which has a U.S. distribution office), it contains no artificial preservatives, color, corn, dairy, gluten, starch, or yeast.

**INGREDIENTS**  tuna oil, evening primrose oil, thyme oil, and vitamin E.

**NUTRIENT CLAIMS**   Each capsule contains 65 mg of DHA, 5 mg of AA, 15 mg of GLA, and 199 mg linoleic acid.

**MANUFACTURER'S INSTRUCTIONS**   Take two to four capsules per day with food or drink. Children under age five should take one in the morning and one in the evening.

## Natural Factors Tuna Oil

Natural Factors "Dolphin-friendly" tuna oil is said to be extracted and refined with an exclusive process that minimizes oxidative damage. It contains no artificial preservatives, color, dairy, sweeteners, wheat, or yeast.

**INGREDIENTS**   tuna oil, vitamin E.

**NUTRIENT CLAIMS**   Each capsule provides 125 mg of DHA, 25 mg of EPA, 10 mg of AA, 60 mg of omega-9 fatty acids, 15 IU vitamin E.

**MANUFACTURER'S INSTRUCTIONS**   Take three capsules a day.

**AVAILABILITY**   Natural Factors' Learning Factors and Tuna Oil supplements are only obtainable through natural food stores such as Wild Oats and Vitamin Cottage.

**MANUFACTURER**
Natural Factors Nutritional Products Inc.
1420 80th Street SW, Suite B
Everett, WA 98203
Phone: 425-513-8800 or 800-322-8704
Fax: 425-348-9050
Web: www.naturalfactors.com

## ULTIMATE OMEGA CHILDREN'S DHA FORMULA

A company called Nordic Naturals has developed the Ultimate Omega Children's DHA Formula, recommended for children three years and older. These are small, round strawberry-flavored chewable capsules that can be safely swallowed or chewed. The manufacturer says that the product "supports brain development and visual function."

**INGREDIENTS**   cod liver oil, gelatin, water, glycerine, vitamin E, natural strawberry essence.

**NUTRIENT CLAIMS**   polyunsaturated fat 0.25 g, monounsaturated fat 0 g, vitamin E (D-alpha tocopherol) 0.5 IU, vitamin A 210 IU, vitamin D 21.0 IU, EPA 20 mg, DHA 30 mg, other omega-3 10 mg.

**MANUFACTURER'S INSTRUCTIONS**   Take two 250 mg capsules per day for children up to 30 lbs and four capsules for children over 30 lbs.

## ULTIMATE OMEGA DHA FORMULA

Nordic Naturals Ultimate Omega DHA Formula is promoted on the basis that it "supports memory and nervous system function."

**INGREDIENTS**   Arctic deep-sea fish oil, lecithin, ascorbyl palmitate, vitamin E, natural strawberry essence.

**NUTRIENT CLAIMS**   polyunsaturated fat 0.5 g, monounsaturated fat 0 g, vitamin E 0.5 IU, EPA 100 mg, DHA 250 mg, other omega-3 50 mg.

**MANUFACTURER'S INSTRUCTIONS**     Suggested dose is one or two 500 mg capsules daily.

## ULTIMATE OMEGA, OMEGA-3 FORMULA

"Maintains healthy omega-3 nutrient levels." Nordic Naturals' Ultimate Omega, Omega-3 Formula provides both EPA and DHA in a 1,000 mg capsule.

**INGREDIENTS**     arctic fish oil, lecithin, ascorbyl palmitate, natural vitamin E, natural lemon flavor.

**NUTRIENT CLAIMS**     saturated fat 0 g, polyunsaturated fat 1 g, monounsaturated fat 0 g, vitamin E 2 IU, EPA 180 mg, DHA 120 mg, other omega-3 50 mg.

**MANUFACTURER'S INSTRUCTIONS**     Suggested dose is two capsules daily.

**AVAILABILITY**     The Nordic Naturals product line is available in health food stores nationwide.

**MANUFACTURER**
Nordic Naturals
3040 Valencia Avenue #2
Aptos, CA 95003
Phone: 831-662-2852
Fax: 831-662-0382
Web: www.nordicnaturals.com
E-mail: admin@nordicnaturals.com

## Attention! Bars

Metabolic Response Modifiers has incorporated DHA into snack bars: Chocolate Peanut Butter and Very Berry Crunch. Ideal for children who have difficulty swallowing pills. The DHA content (from marine oil) and a wealth of other nutrients make Attention! Bars a much worthier alternative to the candy bars that kids usually grab.

**INGREDIENTS**    bar matrix: granola (rolled oats, wheat, barley flakes, crisp rice, cinnamon, and vanilla), yogurt coating (turbinado sugar, fractionated vegetable oils, nonfat dry milk, yogurt solids, vanilla, and lecithin), maltitol, oat bran, date paste, fig paste, strawberry paste (strawberries, sugar, dextrose, citric acid pectin, algin), raisin paste, glycerine, apple fiber.

**NUTRIENT CLAIMS**    210 calories per bar, total fat 4 g, total carbohydrates 40 g, saturated fat 2.5 g; dietary fiber 3 g; cholesterol 0 mg; sugars 19 g; sodium 0 mg; protein 3 g; DHA (docosahexaenoic acid from 625 mg marine oil) 250 mg; grape crystals 200 mg; L-tyrosine 200 mg; DMAE (dimethylamino ethanol bitartrate) 100 mg; PS (phosphatidylserine from 100 mg of soy) 20 mg; choline bitartrate 100 mg; inositol 100 mg; glutamic acid 50 mg; vitamin B1 (thiamine HCl) 1 mg; grape seed extract 50 mg; magnesium chelate 50 mg; vitamin $B_6$ (pyridoxine HCl) 50 mg; alpha lipoic acid 25 mg; betaine (trimethylglycine) 25 mg; opuntia streptacantha (prickly pear cactus) 20 mg; gymnema slyvestre extract 5 mg; folic acid 800 mcg; vitamin $B_{12}$ (cyanocobalamin) 200 mcg; chromium chelate 200 mcg.

**SERVING SIZE 2 oz. (57g).**

## Attention! Softgels

Metabolic Response Modifiers also produces softgels containing phospholipids, specific vitamins, minerals, herbs, and other nutrients.

**INGREDIENTS AND NUTRIENT CLAIMS**   482 mg softgel capsule contains: marine oil (yielding 83.33 mg DHA; L-tyrosine 6.66 mg; DMAE (dimethylamine ethanol bitartrate) 33.33 mg; PS(phosphatidylserine from 33.33 mg of soy) 6.66 mg; choline bitartrate 33.33 mg; inositol 33.33 mg; grape seed extract 16.66 mg; L-glutamic acid 16.66 mg; magnesium chelate 16.66 mg; vitamin $B_6$ (pyridoxine HCl) 16.66 mg; alpha lipoic acid 8.33 mg; betaine (trimethylglycine) 8.33 mg; opuntia streptacantha (prickly pear cactus) 6.66 mg; vitamin E 5 IU (3.33 mg); gymnema sylvestre extract 1.66 mg; folic acid 267 mcg; vitamin $B_{12}$ (cyanocobalamin) 66.66 mcg; chromium chelate 66.66 mcg.

## Neuro-DHA

This is a highly refined fish oil that has undergone an advanced extraction process thereby concentrating the DHA lipid fraction to levels higher than EPA. The ratio is similar to that found in the brain, the retina, and the central nervous system.

**INGREDIENTS AND NUTRIENT CLAIMS**   500 mg softgel capsule contains: fish oil concentrate 500 mg (minimum 50 percent DHA 250 mg, maximum 20 percent EPA 100 mg; 20 percent mixed fatty acids 100 mg, 10 percent stearidonic acid 50 mg); vitamin C (ascorbyl palmitate) 2 mg; vitamin E (mixed tocopherols) 4 mg.

**MANUFACTURER'S INSTRUCTIONS**   Suggested dose is two capsules daily.

**AVAILABILITY**   Attention! Bars, Attention! Softgels, and Neuro-DHA are available in health food stores and independent pharmacies primarily on the West Coast, although increasingly available on the East Coast, too.

**MANUFACTURER**
Metabolic Response Modifiers
2633 W. Pacific Coast Highway, Suite B
Newport Beach, CA 92663
Phone: 800-948-6296
Web: www.metabolicresponse.com
E-mail: sales@metabolicresponse.com

## Gold Circle Farms

Here's something new. A Colorado company called OmegaTech, Inc., is producing eggs enriched with DHA. How do they do it? Marine algae, naturally rich in DHA, is fermented, harvested, and incorporated into the feed given to their hens. In turn, the hens lay eggs enriched with DHA.

This natural, vegetarian source of DHA, called DHA Gold™ is the first "functional food" nutrient to be commercialized by OmegaTech. On the drawing board to be enriched with DHA Gold in the United States are milk, yogurt, and other dairy products. Other food categories are also under consideration, including baked goods, baby food products, and breakfast foods. DHA Gold products including eggs, broilers, pork, pasta, and cheese are already being distributed by licensees in Germany, Spain, Portugal, Norway, Belgium, The Netherlands,

Italy, Israel, Greece, and Mexico. The DHA-rich oil that OmegaTech extracts from the algae is also going to be used to enrich a wide variety of foods, including salad dressings, mayonnaise, margarine, and sauces. The eggs, marketed as Gold Circle Farms Eggs, won the Food Ingredients Europe "Most Innovative Finished Food Award 1996–1997," selected from more than twenty thousand foods. In 1999, Gold Circle Farms eggs were awarded "Most Innovative New Health Product" in Colorado by the *Denver Business Journal.*

Compared to ordinary eggs, each 50 g Gold Circle Farms egg contains eight times more DHA (150 mg) and six times more vitamin E (6 IU).

The same company also produces dietary supplements featuring its GoldMinds DHA product marketed under GNC and PharmAssure labels.

## GOLDMINDS DHA (PHARMASSURE)

Each softgel capsule contains: 100 mg of DHA per capsule (as marine micro-algae oil); other ingredients: gelatin, glycerin. One capsule a day is recommended as a dietary supplement.

## GOLDMINDS PLANT SOURCE DHA (GNC)

Softgel capsules containing 160 mg of DHA per capsule (derived from natural plant sources). Other ingredients: gelatin, glycerin. No sugar. No starch. No artificial colors. No artificial flavors. No preservatives. Sodium-free. No wheat. No gluten. No corn. No dairy. Yeast-free. One capsule a day is recommended as a dietary supplement.

## GoldMinds DHA 80 (GNC)

Softgel capsules containing 80 mg of DHA in a marine micro-algae oil capsule of 250 mg. Other ingredients: gelatin, glycerin. No sugar. No starch. No artificial colors. No artificial flavors. No preservatives. Sodium-free. No wheat. No gluten. No corn. No soy. No dairy. Yeast-free. As a dietary supplement, one to two capsules a day can be taken. Sixty capsules per bottle.

## Women's Beginnings (GNC)

A dietary supplement for pregnant or lactating women, Women's Beginnings contains 100 mg of GoldMinds DHA per softgel capsule. Each capsule also contains 100 mcg of folic acid and 200 mg of calcium, (as calcium carbonate). Other ingredients: gelatin, soybean oil, glycerin, titanium dioxide (natural mineral whitener). No sugar. No starch. No artificial colors. No artificial flavors. No preservatives. Sodium-free. No wheat. No gluten. No corn. No dairy. Yeast-free. It is recommended that 2 capsule be taken each day along with food. There are 2.5 calories per capsule; 60 capsules per bottle.

AVAILABILITY   Gold Circle Farms eggs are available in supermarkets and specialty food stores nationwide.

MANUFACTURER
OmegaTech, Inc.
4909 Nautilus Court North, Suite 208
Boulder, CO 80301-3242
Phone: 888-599-4DHA
Web: www.goldcirclefarms.com

## Nutri-Kids School Aid

Another palatable way to obtain DHA, along with an abundance of other nutrients growing kids need, is through a vanilla-flavored shake. The Nutri-Kids School Aid powder mixes with milk or water to deliver complex carbohydrates and proteins in addition to a wealth of vitamins and minerals and 60 mg of DHA and 15 mg of AA. The source of DHA is the Neuromins micro algae. There are 110 calories per serving when mixed with water. Calories from fat: 10.

INGREDIENTS AND NUTRIENT CLAIMS    Total fat 1 g (saturated fat 0.5 g); cholesterol 10 mg; total carbohydrate 20 g (dietary fiber 3 g, sugars 16 g); protein 6 g; vitamin A 5,000 IU; vitamin C 100 mg; vitamin D 400 IU; vitamin E 50 IU; thiamin (vitamin $B_1$); 1.5 mg; riboflavin (vitamin $B_2$) 1.7 mg; niacin 20 mg; vitamin $B_6$ 2.0 mg; folic acid 400 mcg; vitamin $B_{12}$ 6 mcg; biotin 300 mcg; pantothenic acid 10 mg; calcium 600 mg; iron 18 mg; phosphorus 600 mg; iodine 150 mcg; magnesium 360 mg; zinc 15 mg; selenium 47 mcg; copper 2 mg; chromium 91 mcg; sodium 95 mg; potassium 190 mg; DHA 60 mg; arachidonic acid 15 mg; Nutri-Kids School Aid Blend 558 mg (soya lecithin, Chinese kiwi fruit concentrate, L-glutamine, taurine, flax seed oil, grape seed extract 4:1, citrus bioflavanoids, soy isoflavones [from soy protein isolate]).

## Essential Fish Oil Concentrate 3000/300

The same company produces a fish oil supplement high in DHA, called Essential Fish Oil Concentrate 3000/300. Three softgel capsules contain 3,000 mg of fish liver oil, which includes 360 mg of DHA and 540 mg of EPA. On an individual capsule basis each contains: calories 10 (calories from fat 10), total fat 1 g (saturated fat 0.166 g), cholesterol 6.66 mg, protein <0.333 g, vitamin E (as di-alpha-tocopheryl acetate) 100 IU, fish oil 1,000 mg (eicosapentaenoic acid 180 mg, docosahexaenoic acid 120 mg). Other ingredients: gelatin, glycerin, water.

**MANUFACTURER'S INSTRUCTIONS**    Suggested dose is three capsules daily.

**AVAILABILITY**    Both Nutri-Kids School Aid and Essential Fish Oil Concentrate 3000/300 are supplied through home-based distributors of Rexall Showcase International, a division of Rexall Sundown, Inc.

**MANUFACTURER**
Rexall Showcase International
853 Broken Sound Parkway, NW
Boca Raton, FL 33487-3694
Phone: 888-22-REXALL
Web: corp.rexall.com

## Coromega

Another palatable way of obtaining DHA from fish oil was recently introduced by a company called European Reference Botanical Laboratories (ERBL). This company has produced a creamy, puddinglike emulsion in an orange flavor. It can be squeezed out of the packet directly into the mouth or onto a spoon. It can also be added to juice or yogurt and blended.

**INGREDIENTS AND NUTRIENT CLAIMS**    Omega-3 fatty acids EPA and DHA from fish oil, vitamin C, vitamin E, folic acid and stevia leaf extract. Each packet contains 230 mg of DHA, 350 mg of EPA, 45 mg of vitamin C, 7 IU of vitamin E, 100 mcg of folic acid, and 5 mg of stevia leaf extract.

**MANUFACTURER'S INSTRUCTIONS**    Take one packet a day as a dietary supplement.

**AVAILABILITY**    Not widely distributed but retailers can be found through the company's Web site.

**MANUFACTURER**
European Reference Botanical Laboratories, Inc.
P.O. Box 131135
Carlsbad, CA 92013-1135
Phone: 760-599-6088
Fax: 760-599-6089
Web: www.coromega.com

## New Products

Updates on new products can be found by visiting http://www. lcpsolution.com

# MAKING A CHOICE

So, what is the best approach for someone to take? How much of the LCPs and what kind will be most beneficial for children and adults with learning disorders? From the research evidence gathered so far we can say that a fish oil plus evening primrose oil supplement providing 480 mg of DHA, together with AA and EPA, is effective. At this stage, it is not possible to say with any certainty whether supplements containing more LCPs, or a different balance of LCPs, would be better or worse. Although supplementation is the simple solution for most people, it may even be possible—with care—to construct a daily diet plan of regular food that would provide adequate amounts of LCPs. The same dietary selections should also facilitate the conversion of the shorter-chain EFAs into the longer-chain LCPs. In the following chapter, therefore, I provide information about your best food picks and those to avoid or reduce in your diet.

# CHAPTER 8

# WATCH WHAT YOU EAT

*Food that is good for the heart is likely to be good for the brain.*

—HIPPOCRATES

What should you and your children eat? What should you avoid? Are there any other nutrients, in addition to the LCPs, that can help counter the symptoms of ADHD, dyslexia, and dyspraxia? Although taking a good LCP supplement in and of itself is by far the most beneficial step that can be taken, it also makes sense to adopt a dietary lifestyle that may help to counter learning disorders. This means eating more of the foods that contain LCPs and less of those that contain the trans fatty acids known to hinder the conversion of the shorter-chain EFAs into the LCPs. And it means adding other potentially beneficial nutrients such as zinc and magnesium. Let's look first at the best sources of omega-3s, compared with the omega-6 content.

## FOOD SOURCES RICH IN
## OMEGA-3 AND OMEGA-6 LCPS

As you've learned, various fish are by far the richest food sources of the omega-3 LCPs DHA and EPA. They also provide arachidonic acid (AA), an omega-6 LCP. Meats, too, are a source of arachidonic acid. Even so, the amounts of LCPs in meat and fish are comparatively small. In the studies described in Chapter 6, 480 milligrams of DHA from fish oil were given each day. This is equivalent to eating over 2 pounds of prawns or roughly 2 ounces of salmon every day. In fact, in most individuals, most of the LCPs the body needs are made from essential fatty acid precursors—linoleic acid and alpha-linolenic acid. But where the need for LCPs is high—in infancy, during pregnancy and lactation, and in individuals with conditions such as ADHD, dyslexia, and dyspraxia—the provision of LCPs as well as EFAs becomes very important.

### LCPs in Fish, Shellfish, and
### Crustacea (g/100g of Food)

As fish are the richest sources of omega-3 LCPs, the fish below are ranked in descending order of omega-3 LCP content (EPA plus DHA). The best fish top the list.

|  | Omega-6 | | Omega-3 | | |
|  | Arachidonic acid (AA) | Adrenic acid (AdrA) | Eicosapen-taenoic acid (EPA) | Docosa-hexaenoic acid (DHA) | EPA plus DHA |
| --- | --- | --- | --- | --- | --- |
| Mackerel | 0.07 | 0 | 0.71 | 1.10 | 1.81 |
| Salmon | 0.11 | 0.01 | 0.55 | 0.86 | 1.41 |
| Rainbow trout | 0.08 | 0 | 0.23 | 0.83 | 1.06 |
| Tuna | 0.03 | 0 | 0.06 | 0.27 | 0.33 |

| | | | | |
|---|---|---|---|---|
| Cod | 0.02 | 0 | 0.08 | 0.16 | 0.24 |
| Haddock | 0.01 | 0.01 | 0.05 | 0.10 | 0.15 |
| Crab | 0.12 | 0.03 | 0.47 | 0.45 | 0.92 |
| Mussels | 0.05 | 0 | 0.41 | 0.16 | 0.57 |
| Squid | 0.01 | 0 | 0.13 | 0.29 | 0.42 |
| Oysters | 0.01 | 0.02 | 0.14 | 0.16 | 0.30 |
| Shrimp | 0.01 | 0 | 0.06 | 0.04 | 0.10 |

## Omega-6 and Omega-3 LCPs in Meat (g/100g of Food)

In the table below, which gives the LCP content of meats, the meats are ranked in descending order of omega-6 LCP content, as meat provides only a little omega-3 LCP. Note that there is some adrenic acid in fish and none in meat. Adrenic acid is a very important fatty acid in the brain, and it is one of the fatty acids that were found to be low in the red blood cell membranes of boys with ADHD.

| | Omega-6 | | Omega-3 | | |
|---|---|---|---|---|---|
| | Arachidonic acid (AA) | Adrenic acid (AdrA) | Eicosapentaenoic acid (EPA) | Docosahexaenoic acid (DHA) | EPA plus DHA |
| Venison | 0.09 | 0 | 0.03 | 0 | 0.03 |
| Frankfurter | 0.07 | 0 | 0 | 0 | 0 |
| Pork | 0.04 | 0 | 0.01 | 0.01 | 0.02 |
| Bacon | 0.04 | 0 | 0 | 0 | 0 |
| Ham | 0.04 | 0 | 0 | 0.01 | 0.01 |
| Turkey | 0.03 | 0 | 0.01 | 0.02 | 0.03 |
| Beef | 0.02 | 0 | 0.01 | 0 | 0.01 |
| Hamburgers | 0.02 | 0 | 0 | 0 | 0 |
| Lamb | 0.02 | 0 | 0.02 | 0.01 | 0.03 |
| Chicken | 0.01 | 0 | 0 | 0.01 | 0.01 |
| Duck | 0 | 0 | 0 | 0 | 0 |

## BECOME A CAREFUL CONSUMER

You may be able to improve the conversion of EFAs into the effective LCPs by avoiding foods containing hydrogenated fats and trans fats. This means becoming a careful consumer, constantly scrutinizing food labels, avoiding hard margarines and shortenings, and cutting down on such foods as ice cream, chocolate, cookies, pastry, and snacks—the foods we often find hard to resist.

It is very difficult to completely avoid hydrogenated fats; they are such a pervasive presence on supermarket shelves. And frankly, although it is a desirable goal, there is no evidence that even if total avoidance were achieved the result would be sufficient enhancement of the availability of LCPs to generate a truly meaningful benefit.

Any kind of dietary restraint is difficult for people. It means "deprivation"—giving up the foods we love and have enjoyed for years. It handicaps social life. It is a daily, ongoing struggle. On top of all this, children and even adults suffering from these learning disorders have enough on their plates coping with everyday life. Adding such a rigorous monitoring of everything they eat would be extremely difficult for them.

But let's say you do want to be a careful consumer. You do want to go the extra mile. Take a look at labels on packaged foods and you'll almost certainly not find a mention of trans fats. Present laws do not yet require them to be identified by this name (although the FDA has this under consideration). Other fats, of course, are often listed. As I discussed earlier, the process of hydrogenation that is used to make margarine, shortening, and other products also creates trans fats. The words "partially hydrogenated fat, or hydrogenated fat" on a label actually reveals that the product contains trans fatty acids. Their good features are that they are a source of energy and that they are less likely to go rancid. But these trans fatty acids may obstruct the normal functioning of the nerve cell membranes and they can inhibit the production of DHA, which the brain desperately needs. In people with a predisposition to learning disorders, it may be particularly important for them to eat less trans fats.

The most popular foods that contain large amounts of trans fatty acids are those that we tend to indulge in the most. Look at the following list. The foods at the top have the highest trans fat content. Note that there is no fish on the list. This is because fish does not naturally contain trans fat; however, when it is canned in oil or made into fish fingers, some trans fat creeps in. Fruits and vegetables are very low in fat, so these don't feature in the list, but some meats have trans fat. If you eat less of the foods at the top of this list it may help, but take some solace in the fact that adding enough of the healing fats (the LCPs) is even more important to your health than eliminating the trans fats. And you can easily get the LCPs you need with daily supplementation.

### Trans Fatty Acids in g/100g of Food

| | |
|---|---|
| Hard margarine | 15.03 |
| Cooking fat | 10.37 |
| Soft margarine (not polyunsaturated) | 8.87 |
| Tortilla chips | 4.41 |
| Caramels | 3.31 |
| Cereal chewy bar | 3.16 |
| Butter | 2.87 |
| Cream cheese | 2.76 |
| Vegetarian sausages | 2.32 |
| Scones | 2.11 |
| Cheddar cheese | 2.10 |
| Chocolate bar with biscuit/caramel/fruit | 1.94 |
| Cream | 1.83 |

| | |
|---|---|
| Cheese—Brie | 1.57 |
| Hamburgers | 1.43 |
| Cereal crunchy bar | 1.32 |
| Fruit pie | 1.20 |
| Doughnut | 1.10 |
| Vegeburger mixes | 0.94 |
| Peanut butter | 0.89 |
| Danish pastry | 0.84 |
| Chocolate-coated ice cream bar | 0.68 |
| Lamb | 0.60 |
| French fries (fast-food chain) | 0.43 |
| Pizza, cheese and tomato, thin crust | 0.39 |
| Milk chocolate | 0.38 |
| Ice cream | 0.38 |
| Fat spread (70% fat, polyunsaturated) | 0.25 |
| Pizza, meat topped, deep pan | 0.25 |
| Pizza, cheese and tomato, deep pan | 0.24 |
| Fruit cheesecake | 0.23 |
| Soya dessert topping | 0.22 |
| Cheese nachos | 0.17 |
| Whole cow's milk (4% fat) | 0.14 |
| Goat's milk | 0.14 |
| Cottage cheese | 0.14 |
| Beef | 0.14 |
| Frankfurter | 0.12 |
| Coffee whitener powder | 0.08 |
| Venison | 0.08 |
| Bacon | 0.08 |
| Chickpeas (hummus) | 0.07 |
| Semi-skimmed cow's milk (1.7% fat) | 0.07 |
| Fruit yogurt | 0.07 |
| Duck | 0.07 |
| Milkshake | 0.06 |

| | |
|---|---|
| Ham | 0.03 |
| Low-fat plain yogurt | 0.02 |
| Pork | 0.02 |
| Turkey | 0.01 |
| Chicken | 0.01 |

## ADDITIONAL NUTRIENTS

There is good evidence that other nutritional support may be necessary for children with learning disorders such as ADHD, dyslexia, and dyspraxia. Studies show that zinc and magnesium, in particular, can be deficient in children with ADHD, and it is well known that antioxidant protection is required when LCPs are consumed, which can be provided by vitamin E and selenium.

### Zinc

Zinc is involved in all the major metabolic pathways of the body. It is part of a great many enzyme systems, it is important in stabilizing membranes, and it acts like an antioxidant protecting DHA, AA, and the phospholipids. When an individual is deficient in zinc, the fast turnover tissues of the body such as the lining of the gut are affected. The skin and the lining of the intestine become more permeable and the immune system functions less well. Even though zinc is so important, there does not appear to be any store of zinc in the body; it is necessary, therefore, to take a regular dietary supply.

Zinc deficiency was first investigated in the early 1960s when young men in Iran and Egypt existing on a diet consisting mainly of cereals were shown to be affected. In one study of American men and women, 68 percent were found to consume less than two-thirds of the recommended daily allowances (RDA) for zinc (which is 12 milligrams for adults and 19 milligrams for pregnant women). An Israeli study looked specifically at zinc levels in the blood of forty-eight ADHD children ages six to sixteen and compared them with twenty-eight non-ADHD children. The ADHD children had significantly lower amounts of zinc—on average just two-thirds that of the other children.

Red meats and some seafood are the best dietary sources of zinc. The amounts and bioavailability of zinc from plant foods are lower. Some nuts, milk, and eggs are fairly good sources of zinc, but the calcium content of milk appears to interfere with absorption. Lacto vegetarians are known to be at higher risk of zinc deficiency.

## Zinc Content of Foods

| Food | Zinc (mg/100g of food) |
| --- | --- |
| Hamburgers | 3.2 |
| Crab | 5.5 |
| Shrimp | 1.6 |
| Chicken, white meat | 0.7 |
| Chicken, dark meat | 1.6 |
| Bread, white | 0.5 |
| Bread, whole wheat | 1.8 |
| Milk | 0.4 |
| Eggs | 1.3 |
| Carrots | 0.1 |
| Broccoli | 0.6 |
| Almonds | 3.2 |
| Peanuts | 3.5 |

The Food and Nutrition Board of the National Academy of Sciences has now established the reference daily intakes (RDI) of all nutrients, including zinc, for children and adults. The RDI replaces the better known RDA. These values are not specifically designed for individuals with higher requirements, such as those with learning disorders. They do, however, provide a useful guide until more precise estimates can be established.

The RDI for zinc for "healthy Americans over four years of age" is 15 mg a day.

Zinc supplements can be useful for deficient individuals, but it is important not to take too much. Regular and prolonged intakes of more than 75 milligrams of zinc a day can cause anemia due to copper deficiency.

## Magnesium

Polish researchers discovered that children with ADHD also have a magnesium deficiency, which can be corrected with supplementation. The research group, led by Tadeusz Kozielec, measured the magnesium status of 116 ADHD children, ages nine to twelve. Amazingly, 95 percent had poor magnesium status. In a follow-up study, 50 children were given 6 milligrams of magnesium per pound of body weight for six months. A comparison group of 25 served as controls and were not supplemented. Those children who had the supplement showed an increase in magnesium in their body and a decrease in hyperactivity. There was no change in the control group.

Magnesium is very important for muscle and nerve membrane function and energy metabolism. It is also closely involved in calcium and phosphate metabolism. Deficient individuals suffer from progressive muscular weakness and neuromuscular dysfunction. The heart beats more rapidly and severe deficiency leads to coma and death. Excessive perspiration can contribute to deficiency because the body is not able to conserve magnesium during sweating whereas it does, to some extent, conserve some other nutrients such as sodium and chloride. Magnesium deficiency is very rare in the general population and is usually associated with a pathological condition such as vomiting, diarrhea, alcoholism, diabetes, or renal disease.

Foods rich in magnesium include nuts, cereal grains, chocolate, peas, and green leafy vegetables.

## Magnesium Content of Foods

| Food | Magnesium (mg/100g) |
| --- | --- |
| Macadamia nuts | 100 |
| Cashew nuts | 250 |
| Peanuts | 210 |
| Bread, white | 24 |
| Bread, whole wheat | 69 |
| Rice, brown, cooked | 43 |
| Chocolate (dark) | 100 |
| Chick peas | 24 |
| Peas | 29 |
| Spinach | 54 |

The RDI for "healthy Americans over four years of age" is 400 mg.

There is no evidence that an excess of magnesium can be consumed by eating normally, but it is possible to take too much in the form of supplements. Doses of 3 to 5 grams have a cathartic effect and raise the blood magnesium levels so much that it can cause paralysis and even death. As always, the directions given on the supplement package should be closely followed and care taken not to exceed the RDI.

## PROTECTIVE ANTIOXIDANTS

The normal chemical processes of life generate some damaging chemicals called free radicals. However, the body's cells have defense mechanisms, enzymes and special chemicals, that give protection against free radical damage. If there is a mismatch between the production of free radicals and the ability of cells to defend against them the cell is said to be under oxidative stress. Oxidative stress can damage fats, especially the LCPs, proteins (particularly enzymes), and DNA, causing cell death.

Vitamin E is a powerful antioxidant and, as it is probably the most important fat-soluble antioxidant in membranes, it is a valuable nutrient when intakes of polyunsaturated fats are high. Several research studies have shown that when the diet contains a lot of polyunsaturated fats, the amount of vitamin E in the blood decreases. So if you have a high consumption of vegetable oils, polyunsaturated margarine, seeds, and nuts, it is vital to take more vitamin E. Very often, food manufacturers add it to their products because they realize just how important it is. Whenever using LCP supplements, you should also make sure that they contain vitamin E or other antioxidants to help protect against the creation of peroxidized lipids (rancid fat!) in the body. A good LCP supplement will include antioxidants. Check the label.

Selenium is another nutrient that has antioxidant properties. It is an integral part of one of the enzymes that protect cells against damage. The selenium content of foods varies with the selenium content of the soil in which they are grown. Fortunately, in the United States, the selenium content of the soil is high, so supplementation is probably not necessary. In some countries— New Zealand and Finland being two—where it is low, it is thought that selenium deficiency may contribute to increased rates of heart disease and possibly cancer.

Some foods also contain useful antioxidants. Herbs, particularly those that grow in bright sunlight in relatively dry conditions—oregano and thyme—contain valuable antioxidants. Studies with animals have found that the oils from these plants appear to protect cell membranes from some of the changes that are associated with oxidative stress and aging. Eating herbs, therefore, is an easy way to ingest these important antioxidants.

## NUTRITION AND THE PREGNANT WOMAN

If you're pregnant or thinking of getting pregnant or even at the age where you might get pregnant, you need to make sure you're getting good nutrition. An adequate daily supply of LCPs is essential to help alleviate learning disorders. The importance of nutrition for the health of the baby was clearly shown in an analysis of excellent medical records kept in Holland throughout the Second World War.

After the German army embargoed all transport and food supplies in Holland, there was an acute food shortage in the western region of the country until the Allies liberated the area in May 1945. This well-defined period has been studied in detail for its impact on infant mortality, pregnancy outcome, and general health. One key finding was a marked affect on fertility, with fewer babies being conceived during and after the food shortage. (Women with low body fat fail to ovulate.) In those babies conceived during the famine—and for one year afterward—there was an increase in the number of central nervous system abnormalities and other abnormalities. So nutritional deprivation, even long before pregnancy, has a tremendous impact.

Specific nutrients are important during pregnancy. For instance, extra folic acid—a B vitamin—is needed throughout pregnancy, but particularly around the time of conception and the first six weeks of pregnancy. Supplementation has been shown to greatly reduce the chances that a baby will be born with spina bifida or anencephaly, serious birth defects involving the neural tubes. All women in their childbearing years, even before becoming pregnant, should make sure their diet includes 0.4 milligrams of folic acid per day, according to the Centers for Disease Control and Prevention (CDC). Getting an adequate amount of LCPs before, during, and after pregnancy is just as important. During pregnancy, LCP is transferred to the developing infant through the placenta, with the highest rate of transfer occurring in the last trimester, the period of most rapid brain growth. What's an adequate amount? A supplement providing 200 milligrams of DHA a day will make a great contribution to the needs of mother and baby.

## NURSING NEEDS

After birth, the mother's supply of LCPs is channeled to her breast milk, so the baby can continue to obtain the nourishment he needs to support the critical brain development of the first twelve months of life. Unfortunately, as we've seen, the DHA content of the breast milk of American mothers is among the lowest in the world. On average, babies only get 12 milligrams of DHA per kilogram (2.2 pounds) of infant weight per day—only one-half to two-thirds of the minimum levels for formula recommended by the WHO/FAO.

What should nursing mothers do? If at all possible, mothers should breast-feed their babies for as long as possible. The American Academy of Pediatrics recommends that women continue to breast-feed after the introduction of solid foods, around four months, and do so for at least the baby's first year of life. In addition, take an LCP supplement. Studies have shown that daily supplementation with 200 milligrams of DHA can increase DHA levels in mother's milk to amounts that meet the WHO/FAO formula recommendation of 20 mg/kg/day.

It's not only important for the baby, it's important for the mother, too. LCP supplementation helps replenish the mother's own store of LCPs, heavily depleted by the demands of the baby in the womb. Frank A. Oski, M.D., the distinguished professor of pediatrics, formerly of Johns Hopkins, calls for urgent consideration at the highest levels of the "strategic implications of DHA on human potential." Dr. Oski says that leading health experts and the government should "make the relationship between DHA supplementation and cognitive and behavioral development a national priority."

Everyone acknowledges the vital importance of good nourishment for all women before and during pregnancy, and when lactating. Women with a family history of ADHD, dyslexia, and dyspraxia must, in particular, ensure that they consume adequate amounts of LCPs. While, in general, "eating for two" may be regarded as an out-of-date concept by many health professionals, it's certainly not the case when it comes to the need for obtaining more brain-boosting LCPs in the diet.

## VEGETARIAN MOTHERS BEWARE

While strict vegetarianism (veganism) may be suitable for some individuals, it does not appear to be a suitable diet for those who come from families with a history of these learning disorders. This is because the foods required to provide the necessary nutrients are all of animal origin. Vegetarian mothers must be particularly careful to ensure they obtain sufficient LCPs before conceiving, during pregnancy, and while breast-feeding. It has been shown that meat-eating British mothers have about 6 percent DHA in their red blood cell membranes—three times as much as vegetarians.

## FIRST FOOD

The fatty acid composition of breast milk varies with the diet of the mother. As shown in the charts below and on page 179, strictly vegan women produce milk with plenty of essential fatty acids but with a low amount of DHA. This indicates that where demand for LCPs is high, as in pregnancy and lactation, a diet with a good supply of EFAs may not be enough to maintain the LCP content in breast milk. Less strict vegetarians who consume eggs and, occasionally, fish have more DHA in their milk than vegans, but not as much as omnivores.

**Essential fatty acids in human milk**

**Linoleic acid (LA)**

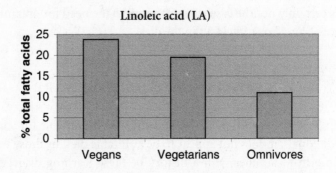

### Alpha-linolenic acid (ALA)

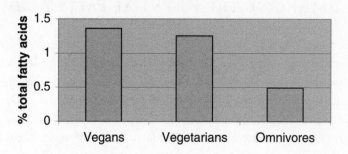

### Long-chain polyunsaturated fatty acids in human milk

### Docosahexaenoic acid (DHA)

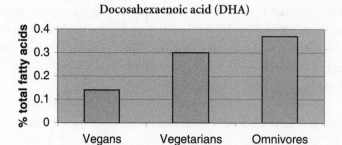

### Arachidonic acid (AA)

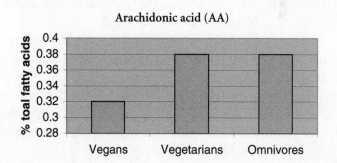

## BALANCING THE ESSENTIAL FATTY ACIDS

For everyone who has a tendency to be deficient in omega-3 LCPs, such as pregnant and lactating women and people with a learning disorder, it is very important not to take an excess of the omega-6 fatty acids. They can interfere with the conversion of ALA to DHA and make the situation worse.

The best sources of essential fatty acids are vegetable oils, nuts, and seeds. Most vegetable oils provide more omega-6 EFA linoleic acid than omega-3 EFA alpha-linolenic acid. The fat in dark green leaves has a higher omega-3 ALA content (56 percent of the fatty acids), but because the total amount of fat in green leaves is so low (usually less than 1 percent), green leaves overall make only a small contribution to ALA intake. Fruits and vegetables have a low fat content and, therefore, provide few EFAs, unless they have been cooked or dressed with oil, in which case the dressing may make a useful contribution.

In general, the body needs relatively more omega-6 than omega-3 fatty acids in a ratio somewhere between 2:1 and 10:1. Like so many issues in nutrition, opinions vary. However, most people consume much more omega-6 than omega-3, so in the food tables that follow I have estimated the ratio of LA omega-6 to ALA omega-3. If the value is greater than ten, then that food makes an excessive contribution to the omega-6 supply.

As I have explained elsewhere, it is important to consume essential fatty acids, and it may well be helpful to avoid trans fatty acids, which interfere with the conversion of EFAs to LCPs. The food tables below, therefore, also feature the trans fatty acid content of the foods. If a food has a high trans fatty acid content (around 2g/100g of food) and a ratio of LA to ALA over ten, then it may well be advisable to eat only a small amount of that food or avoid it altogether. Another strategy would be to consume some other foods to provide more omega-3 LCPs, or take a fish oil supplement.

## Trans Fatty Acid LA and ALA Composition and LA to ALA Ratios of Foods

All the values—except the LA/ALA ratios—are grams of fatty acid per 100 grams of food.

| Fats | LA | ALA | Total trans | LA/ALA |
|---|---|---|---|---|
| Cooking fat | 26.43 | 1.22 | 10.37 | 22 |
| Butter | 0.95 | 0.46 | 2.87 | 2 |
| Hard margarine | 7.34 | 1.27 | 15.03 | 6 |
| Soft margarine (not polyunsaturated) | 9.48 | 2.44 | 8.87 | 4 |
| Fat spread (70% fat, polyunsaturated) | 33.26 | 0.09 | 0.25 | 370 |

| Oils | LA | ALA | Total trans | LA/ALA |
|---|---|---|---|---|
| Canola | 19.70 | 9.60 | Trace | 2 |
| Blended vegetable | 23.20 | 6.50 | Trace | 4 |
| Walnut | 58.40 | 11.50 | Trace | 5 |
| Soybean | 51.50 | 7.30 | Trace | 7 |
| Olive | 7.50 | 0.70 | Trace | 11 |
| Corn | 50.40 | 0.90 | Trace | 56 |
| Hazelnut | 11.10 | 0.10 | Trace | 111 |
| Sesame | 43.10 | 0.30 | Trace | 144 |
| Grape seed | 65.42 | 0.29 | Trace | 226 |
| Sunflower | 63.20 | 0.10 | Trace | 632 |

Note: Only polyunsaturated margarines/fat spreads have a lower trans fatty acid content than butter, but such spreads usually have a very high proportion of LA to ALA.

| | | | | |
|---|---|---|---|---|
| Safflower | 73.90 | 0.10 | Trace | 739 |
| Peanut | 31.00 | 0.00 | Trace | >31 |

| Sweet Snacks | LA | ALA | Total trans | LA/ALA |
|---|---|---|---|---|
| Milk chocolate | 1.02 | 0.09 | 0.38 | 11 |
| Cereal crunchy bar | 4.67 | 0.68 | 1.32 | 7 |
| Chocolate bar with biscuit/caramel/fruit | 2.15 | 0.05 | 1.94 | 43 |
| Cereal chewy bar | 1.69 | 0.03 | 3.16 | 56 |
| Caramels | 0.34 | 0.05 | 3.31 | 7 |

| Snacks | LA | ALA | Total trans | LA/ALA |
|---|---|---|---|---|
| Tortilla chips | 6.18 | 0.13 | 4.41 | 48 |
| Cheese nachos | 2.33 | 0.56 | 0.17 | 4 |

| Fruits and vegetables | LA | ALA | Total trans | LA/ALA |
|---|---|---|---|---|
| French fries (fast-food chain) | 0.09 | 0.01 | 0.43 | 9 |
| Chickpeas (hummus) | 4.55 | 0.40 | 0.07 | 11 |
| Vegeburger mixes | 3.38 | 0.09 | 0.94 | 38 |
| Vegetarian sausages | 1.34 | 0.19 | 2.32 | 7 |
| Avocado | 1.53 | 0.07 | 0.00 | 22 |
| Banana | 0.04 | 0.05 | 0.00 | 1 |
| Olives | 1.16 | 0.06 | 0.00 | 19 |

| Nuts and seeds | LA | ALA | Total trans | LA/ALA |
|---|---|---|---|---|
| Almonds | 10.19 | 0.27 | 0.00 | 38 |
| Brazil nuts | 25.43 | 0.00 | 0.00 | 25 |
| Coconut | 0.62 | 0.00 | 0.00 | >62 |
| Peanuts | 12.75 | 0.35 | 0.00 | 36 |
| Peanut butter | 16.79 | 0.00 | 0.89 | 16 |
| Poppy seeds | 27.20 | 0.45 | 0.00 | 60 |

| | | | |
|---|---|---|---|
| Pumpkin seeds | 21.58 | 0.13 | 0.00 | 166 |
| Sesame seeds | 25.35 | 0.15 | 0.00 | 169 |
| Sunflower seeds | 28.06 | 0.09 | 0.00 | 312 |
| Walnuts | 39.29 | 7.47 | 0.00 | 5 |

| Pizza | LA | ALA | Total trans | LA/ALA |
|---|---|---|---|---|
| Cheese and tomato, thin crust | 0.96 | 0.19 | 0.39 | 5 |
| Cheese and tomato, deep pan | 1.01 | 0.21 | 0.24 | 5 |
| Meat-topped, deep pan | 1.02 | 0.21 | 0.25 | 5 |

| Pastries | LA | ALA | Total trans | LA/ALA |
|---|---|---|---|---|
| Fruit pie | 1.35 | 0.21 | 1.20 | 6 |
| Danish pastry | 1.30 | 0.21 | 0.84 | 6 |
| Doughnut | 5.19 | 0.58 | 1.10 | 9 |
| Scones | 1.41 | 0.27 | 2.11 | 5 |

| Milk, milk substitutes, and milk/dairy products | LA | ALA | Total trans | LA/ALA |
|---|---|---|---|---|
| Cow's milk, whole (4% fat) | 0.07 | 0.02 | 0.14 | 4 |
| Cow's milk, semi-skimmed (1.7% fat) | 0.03 | 0.01 | 0.07 | 3 |
| Cow's milk, skimmed (0.3% fat) | 0.01 | Trace | Trace | |
| Goat's milk | 0.10 | 0.03 | 0.14 | 3 |
| Coffee whitener powder | 0.02 | 0.02 | 0.08 | 1 |
| Milkshake | 0.03 | 0.01 | 0.06 | 3 |
| Soy milk | 0.81 | 0.12 | Trace | 7 |

| | LA | ALA | Total trans | LA/ALA |
|---|---|---|---|---|
| Cream | 0.94 | 0.31 | 1.83 | 3 |
| Soy dessert topping | 9.55 | 1.17 | 0.22 | 8 |

| | LA | ALA | Total trans | LA/ALA |
|---|---|---|---|---|
| Cheese—Brie | 0.22 | 0.15 | 1.57 | 1 |
| Cheddar cheese | 0.31 | 0.23 | 2.10 | 1 |
| Cottage cheese | 0.07 | 0.02 | 0.14 | 4 |
| Cream cheese | 0.39 | 0.27 | 2.76 | 1 |
| Fruit yogurt | 0.06 | 0.02 | 0.07 | 3 |
| Low-fat plain yogurt | 0.03 | Trace | 0.02 | |
| Ice cream | 0.15 | 0.01 | 0.38 | 15 |
| Chocolate-coated ice cream bar | 1.05 | 0.06 | 0.68 | 18 |
| Fruit cheesecake | 0.4 | 0.09 | 0.23 | 4 |

NOTE: All foods vary in composition. Plants, for instance, grow at different rates in different conditions, and this influences their composition. Meat, fish, milk, and eggs vary with the season of the year, the way the animal has been fed, and the age of the animal. As a result, tables of food composition provide a *guide* to nutrient supply rather than a completely accurate estimate. There are two sources of variation in relation to the fatty acid content of foods. The first is that the amount of fat in a food may vary. In some cases, such as fish, it is a seasonal variation; in other cases, it is because food manufacturers alter the amount. Second, the fatty acid composition of the fat can change for similar reasons.

Choosing foods to give you all the nutrients you need and to avoid the ingredients you don't want to consume is complicated. If you have examined the food tables carefully you will have seen some of the problems. Hamburgers, for example, are good sources of zinc, but they also contain trans fat. Nuts are great sources of magnesium, but they have much more omega-6 than omega-3 fat. The only way around these dilemmas is either to hire your own personal dietitian or eat a wide range of foods, including fish. This will make it more likely that you will get all the nutrients you need. But remember, some individuals, for metabolic reasons, have special nutrient requirements. For those who are pregnant, lactating, or have learning disorders, the diet needs more LCPs. If you cannot modify your diet you would do well to take a suitable supplement.

Nondietary changes can also help those with ADHD, dyslexia, and dyspraxia. In the next chapter of the book, I address these life issues. I show what parents and teachers can do, day in and day out, to boost their children's self-esteem, while improving their behavior and increasing their ability to learn. There is also advice to help the overburdened parent and teacher with the pressure of dealing with the learning disabled.

# CHAPTER 9

# MAKING LIFE EASIER

*Learning disabilities are lifelong conditions that may
require special understanding and help throughout
grade school, high school, and beyond.*
— LARRY B. SILVER, M.D., CLINICAL PROFESSOR OF
PSYCHIATRY, SCHOOL OF MEDICINE,
GEORGETOWN UNIVERSITY

Youngsters (and adults) with specific learning difficulties lead
challenging and complex lives. Their struggles are difficult and
painful not only to them but also to those who care most about
them. Coping with the daily frustrations is an almost impossible
task for many parents. Their painstaking efforts to shine the light
of learning into the lives of their children often lead to conflict
and tears as their children labor to do what comes so naturally to
others.

To boost the chances of "getting through" to a child whose
faulty wiring scrambles the usual connections in the brain, the
deployment of a well-rounded, multipronged approach is re-

quired. Recent research shows that effective nutritional support should be a frontline treatment. Supplementation with LCPs can undoubtedly help the vast majority of children with ADHD, dyslexia, and dyspraxia. In fact, some people's lives have quite literally been transformed as a result of finally getting the nutritional missing link their brains needed.

As remarkable as LCPs are, however, they are not a magic bullet. LCP supplementation is probably *the single most important element* in promoting a child's ability to overcome a learning disadvantage, but it is not a simple panacea. The reality is that these children need a comprehensive, wide-ranging support strategy that varies depending upon their specific disorder, or combination of disorders. As I discussed earlier, ADHD, dyslexia, and dyspraxia have been tackled by different health and education professionals, which is one of the key reasons why the biochemical understanding of these conditions has not been fully addressed. Regardless, there is a powerful role for treatments such as behavior therapy for children with ADHD, learning techniques for dyslexics, and physiotherapy for dyspraxics. Caring parents, on an everyday basis at home, can employ some of these strategies to give their children as much assistance as possible.

Of course, entire books and manuals have been devoted to providing practical advice for parents, as well as for health and education professionals, on helping children cope with these disorders. Many of these excellent sources are either quoted in this book and/or are listed in the bibliography. I am not an expert in learning strategies, but because of my professional and personal interest, and from reading the literature and talking with so many researchers around the world, I have gleaned some approaches that many have found useful. There seem to be three key elements to any successful life plan for these children: (1) building self-esteem, (2) multisensory teaching, and (3) learning the rules.

## Building Self-esteem

First, and perhaps most important of all, is restoring the loss of self-esteem suffered by children with learning disorders. This came home to me in a vivid manner when I was shown a personal home video produced by a boy with dyslexia. In it, he describes his condition, his attempts at learning, and, with heart-wrenching honesty, the adverse impact on his self-esteem. Every time I see it, I am struck by its raw emotion. It is one child's story, but it speaks volumes on behalf of all the others who are emotionally (and sometimes even physically) battered and bruised by their class-mates and even, sad to say, by some teachers. It's enormously im-portant for everyone to make a real effort to understand these conditions and what they do to the psychological well-being of children.

There are, clearly, professionals and parents whose under-standing and empathy know no bounds. Through my research and international travels I have had the privilege of getting together with many of them. I've met fellow researchers in many countries—from the United Kingdom, the United States, Canada, Sweden, Finland, Australia, and New Zealand—who share a common dedi-cation; scientists who really care and who really make a difference. Most touchingly, I've met hundreds of parents—including some who had driven hundreds of miles because they were so anxious to acquire information and do whatever they could to help their chil-dren.

In Boston, I visited an amazing school—the Landmark School, which is the educational institution Bill Cosby's late son, Ennis, attended. So many of the pupils there described how they had regained their self-confidence and how they had felt liberated because the teachers understood their challenge. It is in class-rooms such as this that nurturing the self-esteem of youngsters is appropriately highlighted. In Australia, another caring school is the Royal Far West Children's Health Scheme. It provides a home as well as a stimulating learning environment for children who would otherwise be isolated in small communities without the support they need. I also know of at least one dyslexic who gained confidence and knowledge while studying at St. David's School in North Wales, United Kingdom, and is now following an engineering and design course in college.

A confident child is an empowered child. Instilling a love for learning in a child who has already been demoralized by his encounter with the educational system may not be easy, but it is essential. One idea worth mentioning, which I find particularly appealing, is to build a "success book" in which you record all of your child's accomplishments, large and small. When self-doubts creep in and your child is bemoaning her lack of ability, pull out the book and point out all the things that she does well. Be sure to frequently update the book! Identify those areas in which your child *does* excel, and make sure she comes to appreciate that she has other meaningful talents. Spotlight her personal genius.

It may be that she is good at persuading her parents to release more pocket money. She has good negotiating skills! Maybe she can convince others to perform tasks for her. She knows how to delegate and is good at team-building! Sometimes traits that are regarded negatively while young become invaluable assets as you get older. Harvard professor of education Howard Gardner, who developed the Theory of Multiple Intelligences, likes to say that what really counts is not how smart you are but *how you are smart*. Gardner identifies eight different intelligences: Linguistic, Logical-Mathematical, Visual-Spatial, Musical, Bodily-Kinesthetic, Interpersonal (Social), Intrapersonal, and Naturalist.

In virtually all of the schoolrooms of yesteryear (and, unfortunately, in too many schoolrooms of today) emphasis was focused on linguistic and logical-mathematical intelligences. But success in life comes in many different ways depending upon an individual's preferred intelligence. Being able to read and write well is a wonderful advantage, but many peak performers in business, science, politics, and so many other fields have succeeded because of their other intelligences.

## Multisensory Teaching

Seeing . . . hearing . . . touching . . . doing. Open-minded, creative, modern teachers have caught on to the fact that individual children have individual ways of grasping information. Some prefer to see what's being taught. For them to be able to "get the picture" they need to watch it. Others quite happily absorb information through the spoken or written word. Still others need to become physically involved in the learning process. Of course, most of us, while leaning toward one of the senses, still utilize a combination of all of them. Employing teaching strategies that use all of the senses magnifies and multiplies the child's chances of "getting it."

Traditional methods of teaching—in which children are expected to quietly sit still and listen while the teacher lectures—are least effective for children with learning difficulties. Parents and educators need to reach out and help these youngsters in as many different ways as possible. I feel it's important for teachers (and parents) to instruct using visual, auditory, and physical techniques.

In learning to read and spell, for instance, links are constantly made between what we see, what we hear, and what we feel. Yet there has been much argument about which particular method of learning to read works best. I don't intend to get into the controversial debate that has raged in the United States and elsewhere over the respective merits of phonics versus whole language. But as far as dyslexia is concerned, many experts recommend the development of a solid foundation in phonics and phonemic awareness (recognizing individual sounds in words) before using whole language. The reasoning is that the dyslexic child needs to be able to unlock the pronunciation of new words as well as recalling words that he has forgotten. Katrina de Hirsh, a dyslexia expert, says that trying to teach sight words to a dyslexic is like trying to make a crisp imprint in very loose sand.

However, let's not consider one method in preference to the others. Let's use them all! Rather than focus on sight-word (visual-memory), phonics (auditory), or a tracing method (physical), a combination strategy utilizing all three pathways seems most beneficial. TV can be used positively. It can, for instance, become a tool to help a child learn to focus and pay attention. Ask your child questions about the show she has been watching. How did the story begin? Then what happened? What was the conclusion? This all helps with sequential learning.

## Learning the Rules

"Learning the rules" has a different meaning depending upon whether we are dealing with ADHD, dyslexia, or dyspraxia. For ADHD children, a structured parenting style generally works best. It's a style in which parents provide a loving, supportive home environment and uphold high expectations and standards for their children's behavior. The parents enforce household rules consistently, explaining why some behaviors are acceptable and others are not, and include the children in family decision making.

"Learning the rules" means knowing what they can and cannot do from a behavioral standpoint, but parents should be careful to lay down the law using a carrot-and-stick approach. This is usually the only way to proceed with children who have ADHD. The methods of discipline you would use with a non-ADHD sibling, such as reasoning and scolding, don't have the same effect with ADHD youngsters. Their self-control comes and goes. They just can't help themselves.

For dyslexic children, "learning the rules" applies to their need to form a basic understanding of language and the way words are constructed; to learn the rules of how sounds correspond to letters and groups of letters. English is not as unpredictable in terms of its phonological word structure as many people think. There are eighty basic rules in the English language and once they are learned you can spell most words. The few exceptions are, by and large, words that originated in some other language. Dyslexics, of course, like to play by their own rules. I've seen them do it when playing board games. They're not satisfied with the rules that the game developers have created. They want to make up their own.

For children with dyspraxia, "learning the rules" is yet another situation. The rules here refer to the acquisition of the techniques necessary for normal motor skills and coordination. These rules don't come easily to the dyspraxic and require constant, patient reinforcement from the parent, the teacher, and the physiotherapist. A rule for movement that the child seems to master one day can be forgotten the following day.

What specifically can parents and teachers do to improve the lot of those with learning disorders? Here are some limited suggestions intended to stimulate further thought and encourage a quest for more knowledge through support groups, other organizations, and various publications. I have put together a general action plan for all of the disorders, followed by specific plans for each disorder. Because of the overlap between ADHD, dyslexia, and dyspraxia you may well find useful ideas in all of the sections.

# GENERAL ACTION PLAN
## FOR LEARNING DISORDERS

**ACCENTUATE THE POSITIVE.** Praise all of a child's accomplishments, no matter how small. Your child does not willfully intend to frustrate or anger you by acting up, not getting it, or failing in a hundred different ways. Generally he wants to please you, so make sure you let him know when he does! Make a conscious effort to find half a dozen positives every day, and applaud him for these particular achievements. A word of warning, however. It is absolutely essential that you avoid being seen as patronizing. False praise is no praise. These kids are intelligent and will resent being congratulated if they recognize that their peers would not be praised for turning in the same level of work or behavior. This only accentuates the difference between them.

Furthermore, don't just praise—participate. Share and enjoy activities with your child whether it be playing a computer game, taking a walk, watching a TV program, or meeting friends and eating together.

**ACCIDENTS WILL HAPPEN.** Children with ADHD, dyslexia, and dyspraxia are all likely to be accident-prone, so be prepared. This means keeping your best crystal out of sight and out of reach—and using plastic for everyday occasions. When breakages occur try not to overreact.

**JOIN A SUPPORT GROUP.** It always helps to talk to and meet with other parents facing exactly the same daily battles. Discussing how others have managed to cope, and sharing the heartache, is not only therapeutic but also instructive. You know you are not alone. There is strength in numbers. You'll find that "older" and more experienced members of support groups can usually be counted on to provide everyday tips for helping your children. They will also have done their homework and be able to recommend the most qualified and empathetic specialists.

**DON'T NEGLECT THE REST OF THE FAMILY.** Yes, you give your child with ADHD, dyslexia, or dyspraxia a great deal of attention (and so you should),but it's important not to do so at the expense of other family members. It is possible that your other children could become jealous and develop emotional problems as a result of feeling left out. So don't forget to set time aside to let them know how much they all mean to you.

**ALLOT YOUR TIME.** Be realistic. You know your child better than anyone. How long can he realistically concentrate on whatever new technique you are teaching him? Ten minutes? Fifteen? Thirty? Whether you are helping with homework assignments or learning a new skill, allocate short, manageable, and therefore beneficial time sessions.

**GUARANTEEING SUCCESSS.** When you are teaching your child a new skill, or practicing old skills, always begin and end with activities you are positive he can accomplish. Once he has scored some success with the easier tasks, he will be more motivated to persist with more challenging activities. By completing the learning session on a positive note, he'll walk away with good memories for the next time.

**TALK TO TEACHERS.** Offering your help as a teacher's aide or "room parent" during school hours or on field trips is an ideal way to build rapport with the teacher. If you cannot do this because you work during school hours, helping with fund-raising can establish good relationships between parents and schools. Go out of your way to make yourself known to a new teacher and explain the challenges your child faces. But be aware that the teacher has to be considerate of the needs of the other children in the class. Be resolute, but diplomatic.

**COMPUTER FUN.** Playing computer games can be a wonderful way to improve children's powers of concentration, to assist them in remembering sequencing, and to practice eye-hand coordination. Don't dismiss this as playtime—it's an aid to learning. It can also be a fun time that you spend together. And don't forget to mark in your child's "success book" his achievements in the computer games.

**TV TEACHING.** Similarly, don't simply regard TV viewing as noneducational recreation. The dual sensory input of seeing and hearing helps virtually all of these children absorb what's going on in the world around them. TV is very useful in the acquisition of vocabulary.

**OUTSIDE HELP.** Whatever the child's learning handicap, he'll benefit from tutoring or therapy outside of the home, even if it's for only one hour a week. Apart from the advantages of hearing from a fresh voice and a specialist, these learning or therapeutic environments do not have the emotional strains and dynamics of the family home.

**AVOID VACATION PITFALLS.** Parents of children with learning disorders are often desperate for a break, to "get away from it all." But they have to take the kids with them! And that can prove even more stressful than staying at home. Before taking a holiday you need to fully explain ahead of time exactly what is going to happen. Remember that many of these children have both a poor concept of time and difficulty understanding sequences of events, so you will really need to spell everything out. You will need to fully outline the rules of the hotel or wherever you are staying. You will need to physically walk them around the new environment, carefully pointing out landmarks. ADHD kids, in particular, do better on highly active, organized vacations—camping, for instance.

## ACTION PLAN FOR ADHD

What can you do to help a child with ADHD?

### At Home

**NO-FAULT.** Make sure all members of the family understand the condition. Make it clear that it's no one's fault. Don't let the ADHD child become the scapegoat for everything that goes wrong at home.

**TAG-TEAM.** When one parent has reached the end of his or her tether, it's time for the other partner, grandparents, or a friend to take over. Work out a schedule so that you can give each other a break. Single parents will find that it is essential to seek the assistance of understanding relatives and friends (possibly from a support group of similarly situated parents), rather than try to shoulder the entire burden alone.

**DISORDER IN THE HOUSE.** These kids survive with a certain amount of clutter in their lives—and so will you! Learn to tolerate a level of disorder, and don't clean the child's room without his help or permission.

**HIS TIME.** Set aside time every day that is his special "quality" time—fifteen to thirty minutes should be enough. And this should be time in which he gets to call the shots, as long as they're not outlandish, of course. Let him select the activities and take the lead. Resist the temptation to ask too many questions and certainly refrain from issuing "commands," thereby taking over. Be supportive of what he's doing. *Your* undivided attention is one of the most important things you can give him.

**HOMEWORK HELPER.** I have always heard that it is important to make the environment for homework attractive but not distracting, and that allowing your child to use the kitchen table when you are preparing dinner and the TV is blaring in the background is a bad choice! But I'm not so sure. Certainly, it helps to get the physical environment right: a chair that is at the right height for the writing surface, a large enough area to work on, and a comfortable room temperature. But in my experience it is far better for a child to work alongside someone else, perhaps when you are cooking or writing letters or paying bills. You are then immediately available to give help when asked to do so.

Be sure to have all the necessary work tools at your child's fingertips. Having the pencils, paper, pens, glue, tape (and computer disks) at hand can reduce tension. Let's be honest. There are not many adult working environments where there is stillness and quiet. In our working lives many people have to conduct business in spite of a constant swirl of distractions, so why not introduce your child to reality! One of the problems facing learning-challenged yet highly intelligent children is their low threshold of boredom. Doing homework can be a slow process and they get turned off. Allowing music to be played in the background may help many children. Dividing the work into smaller chunks and allowing breaks to do other things can also relieve restlessness. The most important idea is to experiment and find out what works best for your child. It may very well not be what is traditional, but if it works for him or her—do it.

**ESTABLISH A ROUTINE.** When your child arrives home from school, get him into the habit of putting his school bag at his desk or wherever he does his homework. Don't let him play energetic games immediately before settling down to do his work. Perhaps he should do some household chore first so that the homework seems more desirable!

**CLEAN DESK.** Another good idea to avoid distractions is to institute a rule whereby your child's work area is clean before and after his homework. This way there are fewer temptations, fewer seemingly innocuous materials (like pens and pencils) that can lure him away from the assignments that need to be done.

**THE REWARDS SYSTEM.** Provide rewards for appropriate behavior—completion of homework in a timely manner, for instance. Be specific and be consistent. Make sure you have spelled out the behavior that is required and exactly what the reward will be, and apply it consistently day after day. Tailor the desired behavior to be achievable, so that your child can experience some initial success. You can always raise the bar later. And make sure the reward is something that your child will want. His idea of a reward is probably not being given an extra half hour of TV time just to watch the evening news!

One of the most fascinating pieces of advice I've heard is to provide the reward up front, then remove some of the reward if the desired behavior does not materialize. Individuals with ADHD find it extremely difficult to wait for a reward, so they don't persist. They give up. For example, you can have a jar containing fifty one-dollar bills. Every time the homework is not done right, you remove one bill. At the end of the month the child receives all the money that remains and a new "reward round" is established. You do not have to use dollar bills, of course. You could use candy, collectible toys, vouchers for videos, or anything that you know particularly appeals to your child. (This is not bribery! It's no different from a company offering its employees a productivity bonus for targets met within a given time frame.)

**ELIMINATE THE NEGATIVE.**  Unfortunately, no matter what you do, your child is definitely not going to behave all of the time. It goes with the territory. So just as much as you reward the positive behavior you need to establish negative consequences when he's acting up. Say he's arguing with you. Make sure he knows that the consequence is a five-minute time-out. If he continues the negative behavior, he's warned that the time-out will increase to ten minutes. (Don't make the time-out place his bedroom where he may find too many fun distractions. Come up with a neutral and boring corner of the house.)

Persistent bad behavior results in more "dire" consequences such as forfeiting the right to watch a favorite TV show. Plan ahead what the negative consequences will be, otherwise it's all too easy to lose your temper and threaten a punishment that does not fit the crime. You may later feel you have to withdraw this particular penalty, making discipline in general meaningless. To be meaningful, the negative consequences need to be applied immediately.

**FOLLOW THROUGH.**  Don't make the mistake of getting so frustrated when your child is being defiant that you give in. For example, you might be tempted to pick up his clothes after he's repeatedly refused to do so and topped off the defiance by throwing a wild temper tantrum. You say to yourself: Anything for a quiet life. But in doing so you're only reinforcing the misbehavior. Remember those negative consequences that you planned ahead of time!

**BE PREPARED TO CHANGE.**  School psychologist Paul L. Weingartner, author of *ADHD Handbook for Families*, says that parenting ADHD kids is like canoeing down a river. "You need to stick a paddle in every now and then to adjust the direction you are going. You would not think of aiming a canoe in a certain direction at the top of a run and expecting never to make a course adjustment along the way." So, too, with ADHD youngsters.

**BE PERSISTENT.**   You can't expect the ADHD child to change his behavior pattern overnight. After introducing behavior modification techniques, you can actually expect his behavior to get worse before it gets better. You have to give it (and him) time.

**WHEN SLEEP DOESN'T COME.**   Many ADHD children are so "wired" that they cannot go to sleep at the time a parent would deem reasonable. The best approach is not to force him to turn the lights out but to allow him to quietly read in bed, play a solitary game, or listen to music. It is also worth checking if he's hungry or thirsty. Sometimes these children don't always know when they are hungry or thirsty! Sometimes they need to be reminded to eat. A routine snack at bedtime can be a useful part of the bedtime ritual.

**LEARNING THE HARD WAY.**   Sometimes your child will simply have to learn from his mistakes. Perhaps, in spite of repeated requests, he might leave a favorite toy in the driveway. Result: It gets run over when his dad drives into the garage because you didn't pick it up for him. It's a hard lesson, but a more memorable one.

## At School

"School is a cauldron of intellectual, social, and emotional challenges. ADHD only multiples these challenges," says longtime school psychologist Paul L. Weingartner, adding, "Some students can slug their way through successfully just by pure grit, some get lucky and get school staff who understand and are flexible, and some get destroyed."

There's likely to be at least one ADHD child in every classroom. The ADHD child finds it extremely difficult to remain in her seat. Sometimes she'll just wander around the classroom for no apparent reason, disrupting everyone else. When she makes a conscious, determined effort to remain in her chair, she'll probably end up demonstrating ever-more creative ways of sitting. She'll find an excuse (or no excuse at all) to be up and about. She'll discover that she needs to sharpen a pencil (that's already sharp enough) or get a glass of water (when she's not really thirsty) or maybe go to the bathroom (when she doesn't need to go). But hang on a minute. Children with ADHD *are* thirstier, so perhaps the best strategy is to let her have a bottle of water handy. The extra visits to the bathroom that are genuine may be inconvenient for the teacher, but should probably be handled by encouraging her to "be quick about it" rather than "sit tight."

The typical structure of a school's curriculum, combined with traditional methods of teaching and the innumerable administrative regulations, are enormous obstacles for the ADHD child. The National Education Commission on Time and Learning reports that in schools nationwide, time "governs how material is presented to students and the opportunity they have to master it," adding that "the boundaries of student growth are defined by bells, buses and vacations."

Authors Kate Kelly and Peggy Ramundo talk about the physical environments of large junior and high school buildings being impossibly distracting for ADHD children. With hundreds of students moving about, lockers slamming and bells ringing, they say that education at this level resembles an assembly line:

"Students file in to the classroom, listen, take notes, read the textbook, prepare research papers, and take pop quizzes and written exams. After fifty minutes, conveyor belts rapidly move the students and their hastily gathered materials to another workstation in the assembly plant. At the next station, another teacher pushes the learning button of the next subject, and the process begins again." Kelly and Ramundo, authors of *You Mean I'm Not Lazy, Stupid or Crazy?!*, emphasize that they hope their metaphor doesn't offend teachers. But they insist that this is how it feels for the ADHD adolescent who keeps falling off the conveyor belt and can't regroup fast enough to keep up.

The school day is, indeed, a long one for the ADHD child, with periods that seem endless, especially when the teaching follows the old-fashioned lecture style, not the newer interactive method. Teachers talk, students listen! Yes, there are breaks, but not when the child wants to take one, and certainly not as often as she needs them. No wonder it's been said that for an ADHD child, "school too often starts with failure . . . and goes downhill from there." The statistics bear out that statement. About half of ADHD children repeat a grade by adolescence, 35 percent eventually drop out of school, and only 5 percent finish college. A long-term study conducted by Russell Barkley and his colleagues found that 46 percent of ADHD patients had been suspended and 11 percent expelled. So what can educators do to help?

To improve the learning experience of children with ADHD, teachers could:

- Seat ADHD children at the front of the class (under one's eagle eye) and away from obvious distractions (particularly doors and windows).
- Seat them close to classmates who are good role models.
- Structure subjects and projects into a series of short lessons to conform to their attention span.

- Intersperse physical activities between more academic projects.
- Remove all unnecessary materials from the top of a child's desk.
- Let children see an example—and as often as they like—of what the finished work should be like.
- Give the child advance notice that an instruction is about to follow and that she needs to listen closely. Make sure you have eye contact with the child before telling her to do something.
- Give only one instruction at a time. Keep it brief and crystal clear. Have the child repeat the instruction and have her write it down.
- Try to present information in different ways—visually, verbally, and physically. Add color to instructional materials.
- Use learning aids such as computers, tape recorders, and calculators, when appropriate. Interactive computer programs can be a tremendous way of keeping an older student's interest and attention, also allowing her to work at her own pace.
- Schedule the most important learning tasks at the times you know she can best concentrate.
- Give the child frequent feedback on her progress to help keep her on track.
- Make sure you provide activities in which you know she can succeed. Acknowledge and reward the child when she has successfully completed those activities. ADHD children will work to attain something interesting that's within their grasp. Getting an A some time down the road is not their idea of a meaningful reward.
- Give the child tasks and errands that allow her to move around the classroom or venture into other parts of the school. This makes her feel useful, as well as channeling her energy into a positive activity.

- Where possible, allow the child to work in one-on-one situations. Employ peer tutoring, pairing students together to give each other immediate help and feedback. This has the added benefit of taking some of the pressure off the teacher's time!

## In the World

Virtually every parent of an ADHD child has a nightmare story about a major incident in a supermarket, a restaurant, or other public place. Sometimes it seems as if the child has a knack for throwing a tantrum at the precise moment guaranteed to create maximum embarrassment. What can you do to reduce behavioral problems away from the home?

**PRACTICE AT HOME.**   The behavior your require in public should be modeled on the behavior you expect at home. So make sure you establish the ground rules. Your child needs to know that he cannot run through the house, that he must follow your directions and extend basic courtesies, such as saying please and thank you. When you're about to venture into public, whether it's to the store, a medical office, a movie theater, or someone else's home, remind him of the rules that need to be followed. Have him repeat those rules to you so there is a better chance of solidifying them in his mind.

**REWARDS AND PUNISHMENT.**   Just as you have established certain incentives in the home environment, you can do the same when you're out and about. For instance, if you have to take him on a shopping trip, let him know in advance that good behavior will lead to a specific treat from one of the stores. Similarly, make it clear what the consequences will be if he misbehaves.

**AVOID THE OBVIOUS.** If you can avoid it, just don't take your child into a situation where you know you will have to wait in long lines, or where there will be too many distractions for him.

**KEEP IT SHORT.** Similarly, you can't expect a child with ADHD to happily accompany you on a marathon shopping expedition, whether it's for essential groceries or while you're trying on dress after dress. Plan shopping excursions of short duration.

**"BAG OF TRICKS."** Build up a stock of games and activities to keep him amused, especially if you're embarking on a long car journey. Don't leave home without toys, books, and tapes that you know will entertain him. Keep adding to, and changing, the contents of your "bag of tricks" so the novelty won't wear off.

**CHOOSE YOUR TIME.** Make sure you take him out when you know he's up for it. Don't drag your child to the store when he's tired and ready for a nap.

**EATING OUT.** This can be an incredibly frustrating experience for parents! What can you do? By and large, select family-style, restaurants rather than five-star haute cuisine. Provide entertainment. Allow your child to play with a coloring book or a puzzle— for a little while. The best books on etiquette may frown on this, but you've got to keep him occupied somehow. Explain the rules you expect him to follow in advance of going to the restaurant, not when he's actually at the table and already distracted. And impose discipline when you have to.

**CHANNEL THAT ENERGY.** For the hyperactive child, provide plenty of opportunities for physical activities. When it comes to sports, steer him toward a game like soccer rather than baseball. In soccer, youngsters tend to chase after the ball; in baseball, he'll soon get fed up being an outfielder and waiting for a chance to catch a ball. Other excellent activities for the child with ADHD are swimming, gymnastics, martial arts, and dance. Such activities give him a chance to participate as an individual and encourage self-discipline as well as requiring concentration skills.

**THE SUPERMARKET CHALLENGE.**   This is a test of the most noble parent's patience. The supermarket is a treasure house of delights and distractions for the ADHD child. There is the lure of aisle after aisle for him to run up and down. Shelf after shelf stocked with desirable junk food. All kinds of bottled goods just asking to be broken. Numerous other people with shopping carts loaded with products that the ADHD child seems to prefer. How do you handle it? Start small. Introduce your child to a smaller store at a time of day when it's quiet. Have him help you select a handful of items, and let him pay the cashier. Make sure he gets a reward. Gradually build up the size of the store, the quantity of the items (and the rewards!) until you can manage to do your whole week's grocery shopping without a tantrum.

## ACTION PLAN FOR DYSLEXIA

What can you do to help a child with dyslexia?

### At Home

**MAKE A DATE TO READ.**   Establish regular times to read together as a family.

**PLAY TIME.**    Play fun board games that involve reading, such as Trivial Pursuit or Monopoly.

**DON'T MAKE THINGS "ALL OR NOTHING."**    Don't take the all-or-nothing approach when she's trying to spell a word. If just one letter in the entire word is wrong, when showing her the correct spelling note that she got it 90 percent right.

**PARAGRAPH FIRST.**    Teach her the idea of initially reading a paragraph for the main idea and then reading it a second time for the details.

**RHYTHM AND RHYME.**    Make use of auditory memory by including rhythm and rhyme. It may seem silly to sing spelling patterns, but the brain enjoys and remembers them. Alphabet songs and months-of-the-year rhymes can make it much easier to learn these particular sequences. In my own family we made up a little song for the months of the year, emphasizing birthdays. If we were in a hurry the only birthday month featured would be that of our son. So it was always July—James's birth month. Sometimes we would also emphasize December if we wanted to highlight Christmas. The tune we composed was not likely to hit the pop charts, but it served its purpose.

**BLOCK OUT.**    Show your child how to use an ordinary white card with a slit to block out everything on the page except the sentence he is reading. This technique avoids the distraction of all the other paragraphs "swimming around." I have also come across another physical aid, called the Visual Tracking Magnifier (VTM), which helps this process. Use of the VTM can reduce pattern glare, increase spatial effects, and help eye movements during reading. It is a specially designed lens with a horizontal stripe.

When someone is reading text on a page the stripe enables him or her to keep on track line by line by line. As well as with dyslexia, this tool can help people with macular degeneration, cataracts, and optic atrophy. (The company that developed the VTM is CTP Coil Ltd., 200 Bath Road, Slough, Berkshire SL1 4DW, United Kingdom. Phone: 011-44-1753-575011.)

**WORD GAMES.**   Play games such as: Let's think for thirty seconds of all of the words for things we see in the kitchen. Or, let's pair words together such as "hot" and "cold," "comb" and "brush," "arms" and "legs." Such seemingly obvious pairings is a difficult concept for the dyslexic child to grasp, so she needs the practice.

**COLOR CODE.**   When writing, highlight different letters, syllables, or phonemes in different colors. This helps with visual memory. Make the first syllable green because most kids know that green is for go and red is for stop.

**LEFT OR RIGHT?**   To try and correct the confusion between left and right, have your child always wear her watch on the same wrist so that she knows that this is the "left" or the "right." So that she knows where to start reading, place a green mark of some kind on the left-hand side of a page and a red mark on the right side.

**WATER-WRITING.**   This is one of my personal favorites. Let your child fill up a water pistol and spray the water against a wall (or even in the air) to spell out a word. It makes learning fun and again involves the physical sense.

**BACK-WRITING.**   Using a pen or pencil (or maybe even a toothbrush!), write letters such as *b* and *d* on your child's back. She'll feel the difference.

**TOUCH-TYPING.**   The dyslexic student may have cramped or sloppy handwriting. She should be taught touch-typing skills at the same time she is learning to write. "Hunt and peck" will not be good enough for the student who will rely on a computer to produce her finished work both at school and in later life. The great thing about typing is that the machine decides the shape of the letters, so all that needs to be sorted out is the shape of the word. Touch-typing also provides visual and kinesthetic input.

**TALENT SPOTTING.**   Encourage other talents that are not dependent upon her ability to read—sports, drama, arts, and other creative endeavors, for instance.

**SENSING SYLLABLES.**   Dyslexics find it hard to break words down into their respective syllables. Using body movement is a way to have them sense out a word. Say a two-syllable word and have your child say it with you. Then have her perform two body movements to go along with the syllables. She must choose the movements herself. Repeat the action several times with different two-syllable words. Then show her in writing how she has broken the words down. This is a method of physical learning that can then be applied to longer and more difficult words.

**TELLING TIME.**   Dyslexics also have difficulty reading a watch or a clock. Here's another physical learning technique that makes the concept of telling time meaningful for them. What you do is have your child pretend that she is a clock. Position her arms outstretched above her head so that she starts in the 12 o'clock spot. Then have her move her arms around the dial announcing each new hour. Once she learns the relevant positions, transfer the information onto paper.

## At School

In the early years of schooling, special attention has to be paid to making children aware that words can be broken down into smaller units of sound, and that these sounds are linked with specific letters and groups of letters. This is phonics. And it is highly necessary for the dyslexic child to learn phonics.

As the child reaches higher levels of education, help for dyslexics becomes more focused on accommodating their disorder. The usual accommodations are to allow the student extra reading time, the use of laptop computers (with spell check), permission to use tape recorders in the classroom, and the use of recorded books. In addition, there is increasingly wider access to lecture notes and tutors with whom the student can discuss and review materials. Separate rooms and extra time for taking exams are also frequently allowed.

To improve the learning experience of children with dyslexia, teachers could:

- Assign the dyslexic student to a seat where it is easy and convenient to monitor his work, level of attention, and performance.
- Encourage children to help each other. A dyslexic fourth grader, for instance, could help a dyslexic second grader. The older child's experience provides him with a natural insight and empathy. It can make him the ideal tutor. The younger child, in turn, admires and respects the way his "mentor" is coping.
- Peer tutors: Children in the same grade can help each other not only by "teaching" but also by checking each other's assignments for accuracy, and by reviewing materials for

mastery. Cooperation creates an atmosphere of friends working together for mutual benefit.

- Have the child read and reread two or three pages from a basic reader. To develop comprehension, have him talk about what he has just read.
- "Overteach" by reminding the dyslexic child of what he has previously learned or by providing "crib" cards.
- Use funny or even slightly off-color strategies to make odd words more memorable.
- Make sure on a daily basis that the child can see and appreciate that he is making progress, no matter how minimal.
- Use adult helpers. In effect, this increases the number of "teachers" in the room and means that kids with questions don't have to waste time standing in line or stopping work until the teacher can get to them.
- Make an effort to explain things for a second time and in a slightly different way.

## THE RULES FOR SPELLING

Learning the rules of spelling helps dyslexics acquire an understanding of language, and many games and strategies have been devised to assist this process. One of the pioneers, Jean Augur, listed the following spelling rules. Full details are given in *The Hickey Multisensory Language Course* (Editors Jean Augur and Suzanne Briggs, published by Whurr Publishers Ltd., London).

- In every English word or syllable, there must be a vowel or the letter *y* acting as a vowel.
- No English word ends with *v*; *ve* must be used.
- No English word ends with *j*. After a short vowel use *dge*—for example, badge, bridge; otherwise use *ge*—cage, forge.

- *ij* on the end of a longer word, with a few exceptions, is spelled *age*—for example, village, postage.
- Very few words end with *i*. Instead *y* is used.
- The letter *y* has three sounds. At the beginning of a word and in compound words such as "farmyard" it is a consonant and says *y* as in "yet." In the middle or at the end of a word it is a vowel and has the same sound as the vowel *i* has, for example, in "lynx" and "fly."
- *q* is never written alone but always *qu*; *qu* never ends a word, always *que*.
- *ck, ll, ff, ss, tch,* and *dge* never start English words. They always follow short vowels.
- *c* followed by *e, i,* and *y* has the sound *s* as in "celery," "city," and "cyst."
- *g* followed by *e, i,* and *y* has the sound *j* as in "germ," "giant," and "gypsy."
- *all, full, till* joined to another syllable have only one *l*—for example, all + most = almost, hope + full = hopeful, un + till = until.
- With one-syllable words ending with one vowel and one consonant, double the final consonant before adding a vowel suffix—for example, clap + p + ing = clapping, scrub + b + ed = scrubbed.
- With vowel = consonant = *e* words, drop the *e* before adding a suffix—for example, hope + ed = hoped, like + ing = liking.
- With words ending with a consonant and *y*, change *y* to *i* before adding a vowel suffix—for example, happy + ness = happiness, beauty + ful = beautiful.
- With words ending with a vowel and *y*, just add both vowel and consonant suffixes straight on—for example, pay + ment = payment, joy + ous = joyous.
- The past-tense suffix *ed* has three sounds: *id* as in "patted," *d* as in "filled," and *t* as in "jumped."

# ACTION PLAN FOR DYSPRAXIA

What can you do to help a child with dyspraxia? Many of the following ideas were suggested by the Dyspraxia Trust in the United Kingdom.

## At Home

**BE CONSISTENT.** Always be consistent. The dyspraxic child does not react well to change. He can be thrown into a complete tailspin when confronted with something out of the norm. So be sure to keep things in the same place, establish a routine, and be methodical. Remember, no surprises!

Educational therapist Elizabeth Elsworth advocates a regimen of regularity, forewarning, and rehearsing. She told a developmental dyspraxia conference, "Adults can do much to strengthen the life rhythms of children in family life by supporting regular mealtimes, sleeping times and daily, weekly routines. Although change is an inevitable part of our life, the amount of change for children with dyspraxia needs to be sensitively monitored. Giving them advance notice of new situations and even rehearsing what may be required can help these children. When a child can predict and trust what she meets in the environment then she is more likely to embrace the learning possibilities that await."

For example, if a child travels by bus, help him to plan ahead for when he should get off. Use a combination of factors— counting out the number of stops for him, estimating the length of the journey and his arrival time.

**BE PATIENT.** It always takes dyspraxic children longer to accomplish tasks. It's a simple fact of life and they can't help it.

Parents need to make allowances for this, as do the child's teachers. The British doctor Amanda Kirby, who opened the country's first center offering help for dyspraxic (and dyslexic) children, advises: "Dyspraxic children—and the people who look after them—have to learn that there may be two routes to an end point. Both get there, but one takes a little bit longer."

**GETTING DRESSED.**   Dyspraxic children have difficulty doing things in sequence. Layers of clothing can be confusing. Try organizing his clothing for him layer by layer. Start with the underclothes and sequentially identify one layer at a time. Explain to your child's teacher that he will take longer to change into gym clothes at school and that he is not being intentionally slow or difficult.

**ZIPPING UP.**   For most of us, zippers were a vast improvement over buttons. But dyspraxic children don't find them so easy. A clothespin can be a useful ally. Show him how to attach a clothespin at the bottom of the zipper to hold the bottom down while he zips up. An easy alternative, of course, is to go with Velcro whenever possible. Velcro fastenings are perfect—not just for clothes but also for shoes, purses, wallets, and briefcases.

**STEPPING OUT.**   The difference between left and right is difficult for the dyspraxic child to comprehend. Make it easy for him to put the correct shoes and sneakers on the correct feet by marking them inside with an *L* and an *R*. If he can ride a bicycle, put the bicycle bell on the side of the handlebars matching the side of the road on which he should be riding.

**BIT BY BIT.**   Everyday chores should be broken down into small, manageable steps. This way the child will have an ongoing series of little, but meaningful, accomplishments. Don't forget to acknowledge and applaud each achievement. Build confidence by sending him on simple errands.

**PRACTICING SKILLS.**   Once your dyspraxic child has learned a new skill, bear in mind that he will find it difficult to transfer that activity into different settings and situations. Practice the new activity, therefore, in a variety of ways. For instance, use different size balls for playing catch, and throw the ball to him from different distances and angles.

**PICK YOUR TIME.**   Work with your dyspraxic child when you're both reasonably relaxed. The moment he arrives home after a hectic day at school is not the best time to encourage him to run through a range of learning activities. Give him a chance to unwind. The best time? Probably after dinner, and certainly on weekends.

**DO YOU? DON'T YOU?**   Your dyspraxic child is very dependent upon you. Dr. Kirby, a general practitioner and mother of a dyspraxic child, says that parents have to decide when to let their dyspraxic children have a go for themselves (and stand by as they struggle) and when to jump in to help. In the London *Independent on Sunday*, she wrote about how the best of intentions can go wrong. She describes how she was watching her son, at eleven years of age, riding a bike with training wheels. A little boy went up to him and said, "You're a baby, even I can ride on *my* own." Wrote Dr. Kirby, "In that brief attack his self-esteem fell to new lows, especially as it had taken weeks of coaxing just to get him to use his bike in the first place." In this kind of situation, all you can do is help your child continue to try, despite ribbing from other children.

## At School

- The dyspraxic child needs his own space. A work area, whether a table or desk, is better placed in a quieter corner of the room. He'll be less distracted and less likely to knock things over, spill papers on the floor, or bump into others.
- When it comes to story writing, it's helpful if the teacher allows the pupil to initially record his story on audiotape.
- Don't overload the child with too many instructions all at once. Start by giving him just one instruction at a time. Once he has mastered following one instruction, progress to step two, step three, and so on.
- If children have difficulty following directions, ask them to repeat instructions in their own words.
- Dyspraxic children aren't good at keeping track of time. A child's ability to follow a daily schedule can be enhanced by using a timetable containing additional visual cues such as color-coding and symbols. For instance, you could start the day at 8:00 A.M. with the words "Go to school" written in green. At noon, you would write "Lunch," and accompany the word with a drawing of a sandwich or a plate with a knife and fork on either side of it.

## ACTION PLAN FOR APRAXIA

A few thoughts for parents of children with apraxia of speech.

FALSE UNDERSTANDING.    Don't pretend you know what your child is trying to say when you don't. It doesn't help her and it doesn't help you. She needs to be shown what she is trying to communicate is important to you. Show that you care about her frustration and use whatever means you can—whether through gesture, pictures, or other methods—to get to the bottom of what she wants to tell you.

**WHO'S IN CHARGE?**   It doesn't make sense to try and place demands on the child that she cannot meet, insisting, for instance, that she master a word before you give her something that she wants. Don't pressure her that way and don't ask her to perform for others. She won't react well.

**THE CORRECT WAY.**   When you ask your child to correct a word, accept whatever she says and congratulate her for her efforts. If it wasn't quite right, simply repeat it to her correctly so she can hear what it should sound like.

**SIGN LANGUAGE.**   Your child's speech therapist may well want to use a form of sign language to help her communicate. This won't delay her actual ability to speak, but it will give her a valuable means of expressing herself. Be supportive and learn the signs yourself.

# FINAL NOTE

Experiment with the above suggestions. Not all children or adults will find all of them useful, but many of the ideas will definitely work for you and your family. I've included those that appear to me to be particularly effective. When implemented, they should ease the learning-challenged child's way in the world and help him achieve his full potential.

# Putting It Together

# CHAPTER 10

# DOCTORS SPEAK OUT

*To all intents and purposes, fatty acid supplementation is the remedy for children with extreme temperament and attention problems.*
—SIDNEY M. BAKER, M.D., FORMER ASSISTANT
CLINICAL PROFESSOR OF PEDIATRICS,
YALE MEDICAL SCHOOL

We've gone to great lengths to address what parents and teachers can do to help children with learning disorders. We've done so for a very good reason. After all, on a day-to-day basis it is the parents and teachers who are spending hour after hour patiently working with the kids, encouraging them to master and overcome their learning challenges.

But now, let's turn our attention to another important member of "the team" that's involved in looking out for your child's best interests—the family physician. One of the first questions that has probably sprung to your mind while reading this book is, "What will my doctor say?" It's a good question.

The likelihood is that most doctors will have some familiarity

221

with the general health benefits of LCP supplementation. The extremely positive results of omega-3 LCPs in the prevention of physical ailments such as heart disease, for instance, have been widely publicized for some years and many doctors are familiar with these benefits. LCPs are being increasingly recommended across the United States and elsewhere. But so much of the research regarding the benefits of LCP supplementation for ADHD, dyslexia, and dyspraxia is so new that most health professionals may not be aware of it.

This is quite understandable, as the most recent studies—the major U.K. dyslexia trials and the Purdue double-blind ADHD supplementation study—are awaiting publication in scientific journals. Fortunately, I am able to provide the latest information in this book as a result of papers that have been presented at scientific conferences. But let's face it. Thousands of papers on a multiplicity of scientific topics are presented and printed every year. It is extremely difficult for any medical professional to keep on top of the overwhelming volume of studies, particularly a physician who sees hundreds of patients every week.

Your doctor may well ask you if there are any scientific papers supporting the suggestion that LCPs can help individuals with ADHD, dyslexia, and dyspraxia, so I have provided a listing at the back of the book giving the key research studies especially applicable for learning disorders. It is recommended that you show this to your physician.

In addition, in the following pages you will meet doctors and other frontline health professionals who, through personal conviction and experience, advocate the use of LCPs in treating learning disorders. These experts have been in the vanguard of support for LCP supplementation. They have seen enough positive evidence with their own patients that they strongly endorse LCP supplementation as a first-choice treatment before resorting to stimulant medication. No doubt other professionals will soon follow suit. In the United States, the focus of research has been on ADHD children; more attention has been paid to dyslexia and dyspraxia in the United Kingdom, Australia, and New Zealand.

Among the American pioneers of LCP supplementation are Leo Galland, M.D., director of the Foundation for Integrated Medicine in New York, and Sidney M. Baker, M.D., former assistant clinical professor of pediatrics at Yale Medical School. Both began recommending fatty acid supplementation some twenty years ago after reading of their value for skin conditions, and both have treated more than a thousand patients. Other more recent enthusiasts include child psychiatrist James Greenblatt, M.D., a member of the clinical faculty at Harvard Medical School; Lewis Mehl-Madrona, M.D., Ph.D., clinical program director at Beth Israel Medical Center's Continuum Center of Health Care Healing in New York; and Stephen J. Cool, Ph.D., professor of developmental neurobiology at Pacific University in Forest Grove, Oregon.

These experts concur that the best indicator that a child has an unmet need for the LCP derivatives of essential fatty acids are symptoms such as excessive thirst, dry skin, or dry hair.

## SMOOTHER SKIN, SMOOTHER CHILD

Dr. Sidney Baker, who is now in private practice in Weston, Connecticut, has a rather colorful way of explaining the benefits of supplementation. He says, "Take a candidate child with attention, behavioral and cognitive abnormalities who has some signs of fatty acid deficiency such as dry skin and dry hair. Give that child a supplement and you can expect to see a dramatic change in skin condition over the following three weeks. You not only get smoother skin, you also get a smoother child because this smoothness is what we're looking for in behavior and temperament, too."

Is this an appropriate allusion? Absolutely, says Baker: "The scientific mind has become terribly compartmentalized by medical training, so the use of such a metaphor may seem cute to many people, but it really isn't. It's very literal. It has a good physiologic and biochemical basis. We're getting much more flexible cell membranes and a smoother cellular function. At the same time, there's a kind of luster and smoothness of the skin and smoothness in mental function."

But how many children enjoy benefits from LCP supplementation? What symptoms improve? How much better do these kids get? And how quickly? Dr. Leo Galland, a leader in the emerging field of integrated medicine, which brings alternative and conventional therapies together, says that he sees improvements in at least 30 to 40 percent of ADHD kids supplemented with LCPs. The key effect: a reduction in their hyperactivity.

Adds Galland: "As far as clinical responses go, the changes vary enormously from child to child. Behaviorally, the symptoms that tend to be most responsive are hyperactivity; at least that's the most obvious. A very active child or a restless sleeper can see a rather dramatic change, sometimes even in a week." If the child is very thirsty, says Galland, the earliest change that will occur with the right kind of supplementation is an improvement in thirst. That will probably happen within seventy-two hours. At the same time, he says, the child's appetite will become more normal. If the child had an excessive appetite, it will diminish. If he had a low appetite, it will improve. Improvements in skin and hair will take two to four weeks before they become obvious. Changes in behavior, hyperactivity, and sleep can also become apparent in two to four weeks, although they often take as long as three months.

Galland, who has written numerous scientific articles describing the importance of LCPs and has authored several books, including *Superimmunity for Kids, The Four Pillars of Healing,* and *Power Healing*, says that the response is slower in children with learning challenges rather than behavioral disorders. "They're not going to start learning in six days!" he emphasizes. "It's a very subtle thing and becomes obvious over two to four months."

Dr. James Greenblatt, medical director of Comprehensive Psychiatric Resources, in Newton, Massachusetts, has found the same results. He says, "There are some kids who have a pretty dramatic response. Around 10 percent respond quickly, but for the majority it can take three months for the benefits of nutritional supplementation to be seen." In his experience, he says, the LCPs "help with behavior, aggression and mood changes rather than attention," and that providing them to children is "the biological foundation to help their nervous systems get back on track. Without them [the LCPs] it's a pretty shaky house."

Oregon-based Stephen J. Cool, however, has also noted improvements in attention and concentration. He says, "On an individual basis, supplementation with long-chain polyunsaturated fats can have powerful effects. Children have improved attention, are able to focus better, and experience a generally higher cognitive function. I've seen it positively impact quite a number of kids around the country."

Texas psychiatrist Robert G. Wilkerson agrees. Dr. Wilkerson, who is in private practice in Houston, has many potential ADHD children referred to him by the school system. He says, "My experience with fatty acid supplementation has been very, very good. From my clinical experience, at times there are very significant therapeutic benefits. The target signs and symptoms of ADHD are reduced. The children become calmer. They can sit still and pay attention better. They are more sedate. They can concentrate better. There can also be less hyperactivity and impulsivity. It can generally take a couple of months before the patients see results, so they need to persevere with it."

## CESSATION OF SEIZURES

Dr. Lewis Mehl-Madrona, who supplemented more than fifty children when he was clinical assistant professor of family practice at the University of Pittsburgh, agrees that it can take two to three months, but says that in his experience 70 percent experience significant benefits—some quite dramatic—within that time. His patients have been children suffering from ADHD, other learning disorders, or autism with an average age of five. Adds Mehl-Madrona: "In the autistic children who have seizures there has been a dramatic decrease in their seizures. In total, some 80 percent of the children derive some benefit from supplementation and when trans fats are eliminated from their diet some 90 percent see improvements."

In recent years, autistic children have also begun to take up more of Dr. Sidney Baker's time and attention. His opinion: "In the context of the autistic child you see benefits more in the realm of 10 to 50 percent improvement, rather than the 50 to 90 percent improvement that you see in hyperactive children."

Adds Baker: "We need to be careful how to express this, but autism is an extreme form of difficulty with attention. The autistic child, however, has global signaling problems and sensory problems with touch and feel, so any effort to smooth out their chemistry is obviously appropriate. Most autistic children have a dietary history that is simply unbelievable. Sometimes they've lived off potato chips and Coca-Cola for a year. They are drastically low in nutrients. When their behavior and cognitive functions smooth out, how much is the result of fatty acid intervention can only be extrapolated from the children at the milder end of the spectrum. Occasionally, for them it is the total answer. But it is a tougher population to deal with in terms of their behavior, attention and aggression."

As the pioneers of fatty acid supplementation in medical practice, Galland and Baker are both delighted with the new research affirming their work. Clinical studies have now been published focusing on the treatment of coronary artery disease, arthritis, and a wide range of other conditions, most recently manic depressive disorder. "It has been very gratifying to see studies appearing in mainstream journals like the *New England Journal of Medicine.* I've observed these results clinically and it's really nice to see National Institute of Mental Health researchers now proving and confirming the results," says Galland.

Baker points to a major ADHD conference held at Georgetown University in Washington, D.C., at the end of 1999, and says, "When the history of this disorder is written, this conference could be the turning point in medical opinion about ADHD. At that conference there was a lineup of distinguished people and also startling validation that the establishment was finally taking notice of dietary intervention."

James Greenblatt is one of those mainstream doctors who became enlightened about the benefits of LCP supplementation. For many years, as a traditionally trained, board-certified child psychiatrist, he ran large clinics and treated thousands of ADHD patients. Until the last few years, his method of choice was stimulant medication. "But as the years went by I became more and more impressed and overwhelmed with the biological nature of the disorder," he says. "I wanted to start looking at the 'whys' rather than just treating symptomatically. And as I've always had an interest in nutrition I wanted to improve the condition without medication."

## THE BEST ADVICE

Studies in prestigious journals, conferences at top universities, and the conviction of leading psychiatrists such as James Greenblatt are a far cry from the situation in the early 1980s when Leo Galland first began lecturing to other doctors about the benefits of LCP supplementation. "At that time these physicians did not even know what essential fatty acids were," he says. "So I had to explain the basic biochemistry and metabolism and the physiologic effects of the interaction between prostaglandins and cell membrane function. I had to go over the epidemiology and the relationship between diet and disease. I had to give all the basic information and then explain how you would use them therapeutically.

"In subsequent meetings I started getting great feedback. I would run into doctors who would come over to me and say, 'That was the best advice I ever got. It's made such a tremendous difference in the care that I'm able to give my patients.' " Adds Galland: "It's very reinforcing when you see that it's not just in your own hands that it works."

Galland points to a recent study showing remarkable benefits for patients suffering from manic depression as a major turning point in focusing medical attention on LCP supplementation. "This work using fish oil concentrates really garnered a lot of interest and excitement because the results were so dramatic that they stopped the study before it was completed. It's provoked interest [in LCP supplementation] especially among psychiatrists and neurologists."

Sidney Baker, reflecting on his long career, says that he was first inspired about LCP supplementation when he attended an intensive three-day seminar on fatty acids and prostaglandin chemistry. He describes the event as a "gold mine of information—the turning point in my understanding." Immediately afterward he began to supplement children and observed significant beneficial results. He says, "If you improve fatty acid, cell membrane, and prostaglandin chemistry by making more oils available, then the central nervous system will not be very far behind the skin in making improvements. After all, the brain is mostly made of these oils. My interest was awakened very early by seeing children with extremes of skin and nervous system difficulties getting out of trouble very promptly. To all intents and purposes fatty acid supplementation was the remedy for children with extreme temperament and attention problems."

The doctors all agree that there is a society-wide deficiency of omega-3 fatty acids in our basic diet. Typically, Baker, author of the books *Child Behavior, Your Ten-to-Fourteen-Year-Old,* and *Detoxification & Healing,* doesn't mince his words: "From the clinical standpoint in North America most children are just plain deficient in omega-3 oils. If children were animals and were taken to the veterinarian he would say this cat or dog does not have a shiny coat and would recommend fishmeal in their food."

Galland, referring to the same studies I have reported in Chapter 5, points out that the paucity of omega-3 fatty acids has an impact as early as pregnancy, because the mother is the sole source of nourishment for the developing embryo. Everybody, he says, should be doing something to increase his or her DHA intake. Adds Galland, "Our diets also contain excessive amounts of EFA antagonists—the trans fatty acids. I've been warning people about them for twenty years, but it was considered a pretty controversial topic until recently."

He goes on to say that trans fatty acids should be reduced in the diet for three key reasons. The first reason is an increased risk of heart disease. "There has been a lot of research in the Netherlands indicating this and other negatives associated with trans fatty acid intake. But it was not paid much attention to in this country until the Harvard nurses study showed that trans fatty acid consumption was eight times more strongly associated with the risk of death from heart attacks than saturated fat," says Galland.

"The second reason to reduce trans fatty acids in the diet is that they interfere with EFA metabolism and EFA utilization in cell membranes. The third reason to reduce them is a series of independent problems with EFA metabolism that are enzymatic. Some of these problems may be genetic, some the result of other nutritional deficiencies or acquired because of viral infections or other events."

## REDUCING RITALIN

Understandably, these physicians now prefer, in general, recommending nutrition rather than Ritalin. Galland again: "Although Ritalin can control some symptoms of ADHD, its long-term risks or benefits are not known and the drug does not get to the root of the problem. A body of scientific research supports the importance of nutritional factors in ADHD and permits alternatives to Ritalin in the treatment of this disorder. I have personally treated hundreds of children with ADHD over the past twenty years. Almost all have improved without the need for Ritalin."

Galland continues, "Most kids with ADHD do not require Ritalin—it's their parents who may require it! Sometimes the parents of kids with ADHD also have ADHD and can't implement the strategies that are needed to help the child. Occasionally, I've said to a mother, 'Maybe you ought to take the Ritalin and your child will be able to come off it.' We knew what needed to be done to help the child but the mother couldn't hold it together for more than two to three weeks." A comprehensive Ritalin-free therapy for ADHD, says Galland, does require discipline on the part of the parent. He encourages a healthy diet avoiding food allergens and the kinds of additives that, in his view, bother some children. "There's a lot more to do than just taking Ritalin twice a day," he says. "I view the use of Ritalin as an emergency or stopgap measure that's relevant when parents really can't follow through. But all children with developmental or learning disorders should have DHA as part of the treatment."

Lewis Mehl-Madrona agrees: "I have nothing intrinsically against Ritalin and other stimulant medication, but it doesn't make sense to use them as a first line of treatment when there is such a viable nutritional alternative."

Galland, Baker, Mehl-Madrona, and others have experimented with different kinds of supplementation. Galland has used flaxseed oil primarily for preventive purposes, but when a condition exists that needs treatment, he "prescribes" 300 to 400 milligrams of DHA per day in a concentrated fish oil supplement. In treating children with ADHD and autism, Baker gives a wider range of nutritional supplementation. He believes that many of these problem children have food allergies, yeast problems, and magnesium deficiency or fatty acid deficiency, but "supplementing with omega-3 oils is always part of the first round of treatment."

Mehl-Madrona, who favors a combination of salmon oil, borage oil, and evening primrose oil, began supplementing children after noticing so many parents on the Internet discussing the benefits they had seen. He says, "I like to try and keep one step ahead so I began treating my patients with the combination of oils. It is such a benign therapy; I could not see any possibility of side effects."

When possible, James Greenblatt has fatty acid analysis conducted to establish specific deficiencies to supplement accordingly. "My goal and preference is to individualize the fatty acid supplementation. In the majority of kids we are seeing a deficiency in the omega-3s, but in some we see quite the reverse, a deficiency in the omega-6s," he says. As part of a more comprehensive nutritional program he feels LCPs can help eliminate the need for medication, especially if the problem is addressed early enough. "I believe that fatty acids are the foundation for these kids getting better," he adds.

Greenblatt points out that patients need to keep taking supplements. "There was a ten-year-old girl whose mother had independently started her on supplementation. She noticed a difference but then stopped. Within a couple of weeks the girl became more moody, hyper, and irritable. She was put back on the supplement and within a few weeks was clearly better."

## Brain "Comes Alive"

In Orange, Connecticut, Robban A. Sica, M.D., has also used a variety of nutritional strategies in her treatment of more than fifty children and adults with ADHD. "Part of our approach with anyone who has a neurological disorder is to immediately put him or her on DHA," she says. "We don't know how much flaxseed oil gets converted to DHA, so it makes sense to use DHA directly. Patients say they can feel a huge difference. One woman said it was like her 'brain was coming alive.' "

Adds Sica, who has been in practice for fifteen years: "A segment of kids will miraculously improve, others just a little bit, and some not at all. That's why I have an integrated approach. Many parents don't want their kids on Ritalin. They want to get to the bottom of what's really wrong with them."

Exactly what has LCP supplementation meant in the lives of patients? One of Sidney Baker's most significant cases, he recalls, was a girl who had been seeing the family psychiatrist for a couple of years because of her "really remarkable outbursts of temper and rage." The therapist referred her to Baker. "In conducting the physical exam and going over her history I discovered that at the same time she had been consulting a dermatologist for a gruesome problem on her feet. She had cracking that they called eczema but it was really deep cracks and the skin was dry. Her hair was shiny, however, and her skin had a good luster." Baker began to supplement her. "Within a month her feet had completely cleared up and her temperament had improved. It was, in essence, a cure. These are the kinds of stories that are so impressive to the practitioner but just get classified as mere anecdotes."

Says Stephen Cool: "From a clinical point of view there are some very compelling stories and I've seen firsthand some very compelling changes in kids." Apart from his teaching duties at the university, Cool is often called upon, on a consulting basis, to look at difficult cases. One young girl's situation really sticks in his mind: "She was born 'fuzzy,' if you will. That's probably the best word to describe it. The original diagnosis was that she was a very colicky baby but as she grew during her first year she had major sensory deficit issues. All kinds of sensory input just set her off. Everything about her nervous system seemed to exist in a state of irritability. She had some peculiar timing-sequence issues internally. Her sleep-wake cycles were way off. She was not bonding with her mom. It was impossible for the mother to breast-feed her and bottle-feeding wouldn't work either. She had to be fed through a tube."

Dr. Cool was called in to advise. He recommended that the pediatric physician use LCP supplementation. The result? "There were major changes. She made terrific gains in just six months. The general irritability was drastically reduced and she was beginning to interact with people. Her whole sleep-wake cycle normalized as well. And all they did was supplement her with LCPs. They did nothing else because they were really trying to find what the magic bullet was going to be." Adds Cool: "When I see something like that happen you have to say that there is real possibility here. Does it demand additional research? It certainly does, and ADHD, dyslexia, and dyspraxia are obviously the most useful areas for further study. Essential fatty acids, in general, and LCPs, in particular, have major ramifications for myelinization, and myelin has major ramifications for speed, timing, sequencing, and transmission of information in all manner of possible dysfunctions."

As I've mentioned, most firsthand supplementation in the United States so far has been with ADHD children. But what about dyslexia, dyspraxia, and apraxia?

Baker, a former director of the Gesell Institute of Human Development, an independent nonprofit, diagnostic, treatment, and research center, has looked into the connection between fatty acid metabolism and dyslexia. He had a paper, based on a single case, published in the *Journal of Learning Disabilities*, as far back as 1985, entitled "A Biochemical Approach to the Problem of Dyslexia." He says, "The rush to diagnose a child with dyslexia as something only approachable through educational rather than biochemical strategies is rather dangerous."

Similarly, children suffering from apraxia of speech have also not been treated with nutrition methods. They normally undergo years of physical speech therapy exercises. But speech language pathologist Lauren Zimet says that she could hardly believe what she was hearing after some children were supplemented with LCPs. "It really does seem to have a positive effect helping children with their speech difficulties, especially apraxia," she says. "All of the children I treated appeared to experience some benefit in vocalizing or producing a new sound."

Zimet, of Children's Specialized Hospital in Mountainside, New Jersey, became interested in LCP supplementation after the parents of one of her young patients started giving him LCPs. "There were clear improvements when he was taking the supplement consistently. When his parents, for various reasons, took him off it, there appeared to be a decrease in his ability to imitate and produce different sounds. When he went back on the supplement things came more easily to him."

Zimet says that she was open-minded when the parents told her what they were doing. She did some research of her own and began to share general information with other families. She did not go so far as to overtly recommend supplementation, but certainly suggested parents should research it themselves and talk to other parents. "Interestingly, when it rains it pours," she says. "Quite coincidentally, families were coming to me with questions because they had heard so much about fatty acid supplementation through the grapevine. Families had been investigating it on their own. There was a lot of buzz about it." So far Zimet has worked with half a dozen children who have been supplemented who have experienced benefits in varying degrees. Now she wants to do more formal research to measure improvements and see if they can be absolutely attributed to supplementation.

More research is certainly needed and we need many more health professionals to recognize that there is a viable nutritional alternative that can help children with learning disorders. Many parents, like those of Lauren Zimet's patients, have seized the initiative themselves. And, as you'll discover in the next chapter, they are eagerly spreading the word.

# CHAPTER 11

# NETWORKING

*The revolution in communications is just beginning.*
—BILL GATES, *THE ROAD AHEAD*

Networking is as old as the hills. People facing similar challenges have always gravitated toward each other because of their common bond. Caring organizations and support groups exist for every human condition imaginable. And it's no different for the world of learning disorders. Traditional associations, advocacy groups, and support groups are well established and I have listed the main ones at the end of this chapter. But first, let's explore a breathtaking revolution in communication that is enlightening and empowering concerned parents of children with learning disorders. It is the world of cyberspace.

In a remarkable people-helping-people system, information previously locked away on dusty library shelves at universities and other research facilities is finding its way into the public domain. Clinical studies that would never have been uncovered by the average person just a few years ago are now instantly accessible at the click of a button.

Just as important are the personal experiences being freely shared by parents as well as health professionals of all kinds. In many instances, the practical advice of other parents raising a learning-disadvantaged child is the helping hand that makes the critical difference between hope and despair. This incredible lifeline connects parents and caregivers, not just city-to-city but around the world. Previously unimaginable contacts are being made as a matter of routine. Support groups that used to be a meeting of like-minded individuals in one small area can now comprise hundreds of people in different countries. Instead of meeting once a month or once a week, these people "meet" as often as they choose. Like jungle tom-toms they forward vital, lifesaving messages—but on a vast, almost unbelievable scale.

Tap in the letters ADHD on a popular search engine like Alta-Vista and you'll find something like 94,860 references. Type in the word "dyslexia," and you'll come up with more than 55,000. "Dyspraxia" and "apraxia" will deliver several thousand. Thousands of Internet communities are springing up in which individuals and groups with common interests share information on an amazing variety of topics. You name it, there's almost certainly an on-line community discussing it. In two years, since its launch in 1998, egroups, Inc. (www.egroups.com) is claiming to be the category leader with over 14.5 million registered members, more than 280,000 communities, and over 50 million e-mails exchanged every day. When I last checked, it had 152 communities discussing ADHD alone, but only a handful for dyslexia, dyspraxia, and apraxia or learning disorders in general. Some of these communities are small, having perhaps no more than half a dozen members; others have hundreds of subscribers. And there's no charge!

You'll also find, of course, literally thousands of Web sites—a number that is growing daily. These run the gamut from small sites set up by individuals to huge, high-tech endeavors supported by major companies and organizations. It all adds up to a treasure trove of information to be scrutinized, and an almost impossible task for me to give you a comprehensive overview. Instead, I will provide you with a taste of what can be found on the Internet to whet your appetite for further discovery.

But first a word of warning. The Internet does, indeed, provide access to millions of people across the globe through Web sites, mailing lists, on-line conferences, chat rooms, and bulletin boards. These enable you to correspond with all kinds of interesting and informed people. And while there is no doubt that, as in so many areas of life, the Internet is proving to be a boon to people with health complaints and a thirst for knowledge, it is a world that should be explored with caution. Extremely well-meaning people can sometimes dispense misguided advice that may be unsubstantiated, even harmful. Other warped individuals may deliberately disseminate false information. It's a case of buyer beware. Check the reliability of sites that you visit and double-check any information provided.

Teresa Gallagher, who set up www.borntoexplore.org, a Web site devoted to the problems facing parents of children with ADHD, gives some useful guidelines. She says, "I generally use the information on the Internet as a starting point, and follow up by reading any books or scientific studies that are referenced, because of course anyone can make a Web site, so it's very important to be skeptical about what you read. In my experience, the very best Web sites are personal Web sites: someone who knows a great deal about a subject posts information with the hope of helping other people out. When I looked up 'colic,' for example, the best site was by an individual who simply reprinted letters from about fifty parents outlining what they had tried and whether it had helped their baby or not. I found it to be far more helpful than the short blurbs offered by commercial sites."

Adds Gallagher: "I've found the Internet very useful for finding information that isn't getting reported in the press and is not widely known by doctors and other professionals. It's been quite an eye-opener to find out how much of that type of information is out there. It often takes decades for public policy and the establishment to catch up with scientific studies, but by using the Internet any 'Average Joe' with a brain in his head can find out about these studies."

One parent recently e-mailed Gallagher saying: "I just wanted to thank you for putting together this site on ADD and fatty acids. I started searching for natural causes for ADD nearly two years ago. The information was very easy to find online. I too have had much success using fatty acids with my son, now thirteen. He is a different person. Difficulties with fine motor skills disappearing, concentration and organization improving, dry skin improved, you name it. It's a real blessing." Teresa, herself, found out about the relationship between fatty acids and ADHD when she stumbled upon a notice posted by an organization called the ADD Action Group. She did a general Web search and discovered a lot more useful information.

The ADD Action Group, in fact, is a nonprofit support organization that has gone beyond being a presence on the Web (www. addgroup.com). In 1999, it organized the First World Conference on Non-Pharmacological Therapies for ADD, ADHD, Learning and Developmental Delays. Founded in 1996 as a small support group on Long Island, New York, the ADD Action Group quickly grew to become a national organization with fifteen hundred members. It also produces a syndicated TV show focused on providing information about dietary and nutritional alternatives to drugs.

Says executive director Mark Ungar, "We survey people who contact us and find that most parents are lacking in dietary knowledge. Most parents are not providing fish and vegetables to their kids. Most don't get any kind of good nutritional supplement, either, and it's very obvious that these children are not consuming the long-chain polyunsaturated fats that they need. Instead, they get a lot of processed foods and hamburgers. It's an

American phenomenon. We recommend that parents make significant changes in lifestyle and one of the formulas we recommend is the inclusion of essential fatty acids in their diet. The feedback we subsequently get is always that the addition of LCPs had a positive rather than neutral or negative effect. Most parents tell us that they got good results, that the LCPs seemed to have improved a child's behavior and ability to function."

## LAURA'S ONLINE LIFELINE

Laura Stevens, whose personal interest in ADHD was the motivating factor behind the important Purdue studies, has worked with ADHD children for more than twenty years. Now a research associate at Purdue, she, too, has her own Web site (www.nlci.com/nutrition) and newsletter ("The ADD/ADHD Online Newsletter") and finds that desperate parents are delighted to find a source of information they can trust.

"People are very concerned because the rate of ADHD is skyrocketing and the use of Ritalin is off the charts," she says. "I get so many letters from parents saying that they don't want to medicate their kids and asking, 'Isn't there some other way?' I receive horrendous letters. One lady even wanted to give her son away because she didn't have the resources to help him and she didn't know where to turn. She thought it would be better if she left him with family services. Another woman said she could never take her kid out in public with her because his behavior was so abnormal. It's not unusual to have a letter saying, 'My son has been expelled from school four times and the next time it's going to be permanent. I'm desperate.' The letters are just heartbreaking."

Many of these children, says Stevens, author of *12 Effective Ways to Help Your ADD/ADHD Child*, not only have ADHD, but they also have behavior abnormalities such as conduct disorder or oppositional defiance disorder. Or they might have depression or problems with their motor skills. "So these kids not only have the curse of ADHD, they have other problems that may make it very difficult to parent them," she says. "Fortunately, there is a groundswell of scientific interest in nutritional answers and more studies are being conducted."

## RESEARCH UPDATE

Clinical child psychologist and research professor David Rabiner of Duke University started a subscription newsletter "ADHD Research Update" in August of 1997 that is now distributed to more than sixteen thousand parents and professionals. "My primary goal was to provide parents with access to up-to-date research information on ADHD so they could make well-informed decisions about helping their child," he says. "Basically, without the Internet, there would have been no way for me to distribute this information to parents. I could not have afforded to publicize my newsletter except via the Net, nor could I have sent out print copies to everyone who requested them."

## YOUR HUMAN GUIDE

The Internet's only network of sites led by expert human guides—www.about.com—boasts a wealth of information about ADHD. The ADHD "human guide," Bob Seay, is not a medical practitioner but brings to the table his personal experience as an adult with ADHD. Undiagnosed until his mid-thirties, Seay's chatty, sometimes blunt, style of writing presents a refreshing picture of life with ADHD.

One sample: Seay wrote an article about *Time* magazine

naming Albert Einstein "Person of the Century." Headlined "Albert Einstein—He's One of Us!!!," he commented: "Einstein has been a folk hero for the ADD community for some time. While never diagnosed, comparing Einstein and ADD behaviors makes for an intriguing study. An almost cultic following has emerged including ADD tee shirts bearing Einstein's image. Of all of the famous people who may have been ADD, Einstein is by far the most popular. He may be a Cultural Icon, but he's our Cultural Icon!"

Later in the same article: "Some have speculated that were he alive today, Einstein would have been put on Ritalin to manage his ADD. . . . If this had been the case, how would our world be different today. Would Einstein still be an Einstein? . . . Are we medicating away the geniuses? Or would medications have helped Einstein?" Bob's Web site (www.add.about.com) is a mine of information and has many useful links. Bob's regular free newsletter, "ADDed Stuff," also provides information on the latest research as well as the "politics" of ADHD.

## HELP FROM HALLOWELL

Also well worth a visit is the Web site of Edward M. Hallowell, M.D., co-author of the best-sellers *Driven To Distraction* and *Answers to Distraction* (www.drhallowell.com). Twenty years in private practice, and being an instructor at Harvard Medical School, give Dr. Hallowell the knowledge and experience to enable him to speak authoritatively on the subject of ADD and learning disorders. The fact that he, too, has both ADD and dyslexia gives him that extra personal understanding.

# THE APRAXIA DIALOG

Internet information about apraxia and dyspraxia came to me thanks to Donna Marucci of Pittsburgh, Pennsylvania, an Internet-savvy grandmother who variously describes herself as the "granny on a mission" and the "granny from hell." She is certainly one determined lady who refused to leave any stone unturned when her grandson Jesse's learning handicap was diagnosed as apraxia.

"Our reaction was 'apraxi-what?' " remembers Marucci, asking, "So where do people go when they are given a diagnosis most people have never heard of?" Answering her own question she says that today the Internet is the place to go. She simply typed the word "apraxia" on a search engine and discovered the apraxia-kids Web site and listserv (www.apraxia-kids.org). In no time, Marucci was communicating with parents around the world. "Through information gained from others on the list, I was given guidance as to what type of medical doctors needed to be seen and what steps to take to ensure proper treatment. We were so thankful for this resource," she says.

The Web site and listserv that the "granny on a mission" had found was started by Sharon Gretz, herself the mother of an apraxic child. When Gretz's child was diagnosed, she began to research the subject and ran into a brick wall. She was not able to locate any information aimed at parents. All she could find was professional literature. She decided, therefore, to fill the void so that other "worried and struggling parents" would have an easier time.

The apraxia-kids listserv was launched in January 1997 with just a handful of subscribers. Today the list has over fifteen hundred subscribers and continues to grow. With the help of another parent, Gina Mikel, a companion Web site followed in May 1997 and is used extensively by parents as well as speech language clinicians, educators, and other professionals. It is now widely recognized as the most extensive and comprehensive place for information about developmental apraxia of speech that is on the World Wide Web. Says Donna Marucci, "When you did a search on apraxia five years ago nothing came up. Now there are volumes of information. We owe Sharon Gretz so much. So many parents will be eternally grateful to her for having started this listserv and Web site. It has provided answers and support when everything looked so bleak and dark."

During 1999 the subject of LCPs began to be discussed on the listserv more and more frequently, at times dominating the dialog. Another mother, Melanie Foutch, decided therefore to set up another list to specifically discuss nutritional supplements and diet, and this was the beginning of the Speech Diet list (www. egroups.com/groups/SpeechDiet). Says Foutch: "With a dedicated forum such as the Speech Diet list, parents are able to share their experiences in greater detail. . . . One parent can only read and research a limited amount of material. One parent can only experiment with a limited amount of supplements and can only see the results in her child. By having a forum for exchanging information, hundreds of parents are able to share and catalog their results, allowing everyone to become more informed and educated. If it were not for the communities (listservs, mailing lists, etc.) on the Internet, I would not have known about the success of fatty acid supplementation, nor would I have been exposed to the hundreds of parent testimonials about its benefits. The success stories were the deciding factor in our choice to give our child fatty acid supplements, more so than any research literature on the subject."

Marucci continues the story about the development of the Speech Diet list: "Before we knew it, there were over 160 members. We have members whose children have various learning disorders or disabilities. . . . We've researched every source of information available and we're a real team, each helping the other giving guidance and passing on information. The Internet has been a lifesaver for my family, and many others. The Internet has put us in contact with researchers, chemists, nutritionists and many other experts, as well as many parents who are in similar situations with their own children.

"Most of the members of the Speech Diet list supplement their children's diets with some form of fatty acids, and so the discussion continues. The most common story is how every parent is given 'the wait.' They are told that their child is 'just slow,' that 'boys are slower than girls,' that 'Einstein never talked until he was four years old.' Most of us feel that there needs to be assessment much sooner and consideration given to the fact that some children are not 'just slow.' "

List owner Melanie Foutch's son was fortunately recognized as having a problem earlier than most. She says, "At nineteen months it was determined that he had a speech and language delay of unknown origin. After months of therapy and minimal results, I heard about fatty acid supplements and decided to try them. We saw excellent progress, beginning about three weeks after we started supplementing him. His speech and language seem to have been jump-started. Progress continued steadily, not only in speech issues, but behavioral issues as well. He has seemed much more organized and focused."

## TALKING TO OTHERS

Other useful resources on the Internet include mailing lists, conferences, and bulletin boards. With these you can post your own questions and observations and respond to other people's messages at your own convenience. However, remember that you need to carefully assess any information you may receive as the quality and accuracy can vary enormously, and very often you don't really know to whom you are "talking."

## Usenet Groups

There's a growing number of Internet newsgroups called Usenet, focusing on ADHD, dyslexia, and dyspraxia, and you'll find people asking questions, giving answers, and delivering unsolicited opinions on every aspect of these disorders. One well-known and busy group is alt.support.attn-deficit. Also look for alt.support. dyslexia and alt.support.dyspraxia. You can access them through www.deja.com/usenet, which claims to be the largest "discussion service" including Usenet, newsgroups, and other forums. If you have any difficulty accessing such groups, your internet service provider (ISP) should be able to provide assistance.

## Chat Rooms

In chat rooms you can "talk live" to other people. You may well find that there are overlaps in conversation and that people frequently veer off-topic, but they do allow for real communication, often giving you the opportunity to pose questions to experts. The organization Children and Adults with Attention Deficit Disorder (CHADD) has one at http://chat.chaddonline.org. An about.com chat room can be found at http://add.about.com/mpchat.htm.

## Dyslexia Online Magazine

A magazine containing articles about dyslexia for both parents of children with dyslexia and adults with dyslexia. www.dyslexia-magazine.com

## Dyslexia WebRing

A collection of more than twenty different sites about dyslexia. Some are personal stories of people struggling with dyslexia; some are commercial sites. Go to www.webring.org and enter dyslexia as the key word.

# KEY WEB SITES—A MINI DIRECTORY

Most of the major support organizations—such as the International Dyslexia Association, Children and Adults with Attention-Deficit/Hyperactivity Disorder, and the National Attention Deficit Disorder Association—all have their own Web sites. Here is a key list of Internet connections followed by more detailed information about various organizations. With regard to the Web sites, it is important to note that the Internet is a volatile, ever-changing medium. Well-meaning people often start a Web site or discussion group and when their enthusiasm wanes do not maintain them. I have, therefore, endeavored to focus on established presences that are likely to remain in existence.

## Learning Disabilities

For excellent information about learning disorders in general look to the Web site at www.ldonline.org, picked by *Access Internet* magazine as one of the best Web sites of 1999. Put together by the Learning Project at WETA, the public broadcasting station in Washington, D.C., it's the official Web site of the Coordinated

Campaign for Learning Disabilities, an organization that pro-
motes public awareness of learning disabilities. The site contains a
lot of in-depth information. There is also an excellent free monthly
newsletter—"The LD Online Report"—as well as bulletin boards
and chat rooms with visiting experts.

## Contacting Dr. Stordy

I have my own Web site and e-zine at www.drstordy.com.
    You can e-mail to: info@www.drstordy.com. The site is devoted
to providing the very latest information including scientific research
on ADHD, dyslexia, dyspraxia, apraxia, and related disorders.

## ADHD

### "THE ADD/ADHD ONLINE NEWSLETTER"

This is a publication designed to help children and adults with
ADHD authored by researcher Laura Stevens of Purdue University. www.nlci.com/nutrition

### "ADHD RESEARCH UPDATE"

A subscription newsletter sent to parents and professionals interested in keeping up with the latest ADHD research, produced by
David Rabiner, Ph.D., of Duke University. Dr. Rabiner also provides a free ADHD Monitoring System designed to help parents
monitor their children's progress at school. Free samples of the
newsletter can be obtained from: www.helpforadd.com

## YOUR HUMAN GUIDE

Check out Bob Seay's Web site, e-zine, extensive list of resources and articles, as well as on-line forums. Well worth a visit. www.add.about.com

## "ADDITUDE"

An on-line magazine, sister publication to a print magazine of the same name that launched in June 2000. *ADDitude* claims to be America's first independent consumer and lifestyle magazine for adults and children with attention deficits and related learning disabilities. Among its goals: destigmatizing ADD by increasing public awareness through education and information. The on-line magazine also has its own discussion board. www.additudemag.com

## "THE ADD-ADHD GAZETTE"

From the United Kingdom, Gail Miller has been publishing *The ADD/ADHD Gazette* since early 1999 and within a year had amassed 2,500 subscribers. The free e-zine concentrates on education, legislation, books, research, and behavior management. It also lists e-mail discussion groups and forums. http://home.freeuk.net/theadhdgazette

## WORTH CHECKING OUT

A British-based Web site full of good information:
    www.adders.org
Another useful site with a newsletter, articles, and message
    board: www.adhdnews.com

A site that describes itself as "a virtual neighborhood
consolidating in one place information and resources
related to ADHD and learning disorders" can be found at
www.oneaddplace.com

## MAJOR ADHD ORGANIZATIONS

Children and Adults with Attention-Deficit/Hyperactivity
Disorder: www.chadd.org
National Attention Deficit Disorder Association: www.add.org

# Dyslexia

## HELLO FRIEND

The Hello Friend Web site is definitely one you should explore. It
was established by the nonprofit Ennis William Cosby Foundation and contains a tremendous amount of motivating and useful
information. www.hellofriend.org

## DON WINKLER

Visit the Web site of Donald A. Winkler, chairman and CEO of the
Ford Motor Credit Company, the world's largest automotive
finance company. Don, who has dyslexia and other learning
disabilities, is a board member of the International Dyslexia
Association. Read his inspiring success story, learn about his
Breakthrough Leadership Process, and check out his suggested
resources. www.cyberwink.com

## DYSLEXICS.NET

This is a Web site offering a broad spectrum of information about dyslexia. There are a large number of articles about the disorder, plus lists of chat rooms, forums, discussion boards, and newsgroups. It also lists various organizations and commercial programs. www.dyslexics.net

## MAJOR DYSLEXIA ORGANIZATIONS

The International Dyslexia Association: www.interdys.org
British Dyslexia Association: www.bda-dyslexia.org.uk
World Dyslexia Network Foundation (with links to many other sites): www.surrey.ac.uk/Psychology/WDNF/front.html

# Dyspraxia/Apraxia

## APRAXIA-KIDS

The apraxia-kids list connects parents and professionals across the world. You should visit the Web site first at: www.apraxia-kids.org and then follow the directions to subscribe to this very active list.

## SPEECH DIET

This is the list in which parents specifically discuss the benefits of LCPs and other nutritional interventions for children with apraxia of speech. Many of the extremely well-informed parents on the apraxia Speech Diet list were most helpful to me. Subscribe by going to: www.egroups.com/group/SpeechDiet

# Online Communities

Check out www.eGroups.com and see which lists appeal to you.
You'll find several that specifically address the issue of nutritional
supplementation and dietary intervention.

# Other Online Resources

## INTERNET SPECIAL EDUCATION RESOURCES (ISER)

A kind of online yellow pages, ISER is a nationwide directory of
professionals who serve the learning disabilities and special education communities. It helps parents and caregivers find local
special education professionals to help with learning disabilities
and attention deficit disorder assessment, therapy, advocacy, and
other special needs. ISER is at www.iser.com

## ALL KINDS OF MINDS

This is the Web site of the nonprofit institute of the same name that
"helps families, educators, and clinicians understand why children
are struggling in school and provides practical strategies to help
them become successful learners." Founded by eminent pediatric
expert Dr. Mel Levine, All Kinds of Minds has well-researched, authoritative information as well as discussion groups and an online
newsletter. www.allkindsofminds.org

## COORDINATED CAMPAIGN FOR LEARNING DISABILITIES

This is the comprehensive, award-winning Web site I mentioned earlier in the chapter. A gold mine of good, solid information. www.ldonline.org

## LD RESOURCES

This detailed site put together by Richard Wanderman contains a host of resources and links to other sites, as well as contact information for national and regional organizations, conferences, and schools. It also includes a host of interesting articles. www.ldresources.com

## MENTAL HEALTH NET

Claimed to be "the oldest and largest online mental health directory guide and community," this site is a compendium of data and resources. It lists and rates Web sites on specific disorders with a "thumbs up" or "thumbs down," based on input from visitors: http://mentalhelp.net To go directly to the ADHD section: http://adhd.mentalhelp.net/

## SCHWAB FOUNDATION FOR LEARNING

The Web site of the foundation started by discount brokerage pioneer Charles R. Schwab and his wife, Helen O'Neill Schwab, provides wide-ranging and comprehensive information for parents and educators helping kids with learning differences. The foundation's mission grew out of Charles Schwab's lifelong struggle with dyslexia and the frustration he faced trying to find help for his son who inherited the disorder. Its staff provides personal responses. www.schwablearning.org

## SPECIAL EDUCATION RESOURCES ON THE INTERNET (SERI)

SERI is a large collection of sites of interest to those involved in the fields of special education. It is hosted at Hood College in Frederick, Maryland. www.hood.edu/seri

# RESOURCES

# ADHD

ADD Anonymous
P.O. Box 421227
San Diego, CA 92142-1227
Phone: 619-560-6190
Fax: 619-560-6190
E-mail: addanon@aol.com
Founded in 1996 to carry the message of the twelve steps to adults with attention deficit disorder. There are ten affiliated groups. Assistance provided in starting groups.

Attention Deficit Disorder Association (ADDA)
9930 Johnnycake Ridge Road, Suite 3E
Mentor, OH 44060
Phone: 216-350-9595 or 800-487-2282
Fax: 216-350-0223
E-mail: natladda@aol.com
ADDA supplies educational resources on attention disorders

to individuals and support organizations. The organization has a special interest in the needs of adults with ADHD. It has a newsletter, produces information and referrals, and hosts a national conference and speakers bureau.

ADDIEN ADDult Information Exchange Network
P.O. Box 1991
Ann Arbor, MI 48106
Phone: 734-426-1659
Fax: 734-426-0116
Web: www.addien.org
E-mail: addien@aol.com

An organization largely focused on providing support to adults with ADHD. Holds an annual conference.

Attention Deficit Information Network, Inc. (AD-IN)
475 Hillside Avenue
Needham, MA 02194
Phone: 781-455-9895
Fax: 781-444-5466
Web: www.addinfonetwork.com
E-mail: adin@gis.net

AD-IN is a nonprofit volunteer organization that was founded in 1984. It offers support and information to families of children and adults with ADD, as well as to professionals. There are twenty-five chapters throughout the country. AD-IN also presents conferences and workshops for parents and professionals on current issues, research, and treatment options.

ADD Action Group
175 West 72nd Street, 2nd floor
New York, NY 10023

Phone: 212-769-2457
Fax: 212-769-2457
Web: www.addgroup.org
E-mail: addinquir@aol.com

The ADD Action group is a nonprofit organization that helps people find alternative, nondrug solutions for attention deficit disorder, learning differences, dyslexia, and autism. The group has a monthly newsletter and provides information and referrals, phone support, conferences, literature, and advocacy.

Children and Adults with Attention Deficit Disorder
(CHADD)
8181 Professional Place, Suite 201
Landover, MD 20785
Phone: 301-306-7070 or 800-233-4050
Fax: 301-306-7090
Web: www.chadd.org
E-mail: national@chadd.org

Founded in 1987, CHADD is a national and international nonprofit support organization that provides information, sponsors conferences, and holds meetings and support groups. With over 32,000 members and 500 chapters throughout the United States, it is the leading organization of its kind.

Feingold Association of the United States
Box 6550
Alexandria, VA 22306
Phone: 703-768-3287 or 808-321-3287
Web: www.feingold.org

An organization of families and professionals, the nonprofit Feingold Association is dedicated to helping children and adults apply dietary techniques for better behavior, learning, and health. The organization provides newsletters, food guides, telephone, and e-mail help lines. There are also group support meetings in some parts of the country.

The National Attention Deficit Disorder Association
1788 Second Street, Suite 200
Highland Park, IL 60035
Phone: 847-432-ADDA
Fax: 847-432-5874
Web: www.add.org
E-mail: mail@add.org

A national nonprofit organization focusing on adults and families, ADDA provides referrals to local support groups, holds national conferences and symposiums, and offers materials on ADHD and related issues.

## Dyslexia

Dyslexia Research Institute, Inc.
5746 Centerville Road
Tallahassee, FL 32308
Phone: 850-893-2216
Fax: 850-893-2440
Web: www. dyslexia-add.org
E-mail: dri@dyslexia-add.org

Since 1975, the goal of the Dyslexia Research Institute, Inc., has been to change the perception of learning differences, specifically in the area of dyslexia and ADHD. The organization supplies parenting information, adult education, advocacy, and consultation as well as research and development resources.

Hello Friend/Ennis William Cosby Foundation
P.O. Box 4061
Santa Monica, CA 90411

Web: www.hellofriend.org

Established by Bill and Camille Cosby to fulfill the goals and dreams of their son, the foundation was formed in early 1997 as a public, nonprofit organization. It is dedicated to helping all people with dyslexia and language-based learning differences reach their full potential.

International Dyslexia Association
(formerly The Orton Dyslexia Society)
Chester Building, Suite 382
8600 La Salle Road
Baltimore, MD 21286-2044
Phone: 410-296-0232 or 800-222-3123 (ABCD123)
Fax: 410-321-5069
Web: www.interdys.org
E-mail: info@interdys.org

The International Dyslexia Association is a nonprofit, scientific, and educational organization dedicated to the study and treatment of dyslexia. The IDA was first established nearly fifty years ago to continue the pioneering work of Dr. Samuel T. Orton. There are chapters throughout the United States offering information and support meetings to its more than eleven thousand members.

Recordings for the Blind and Dyslexic (RFB&D)
20 Roszel Road
Princeton, NJ 08540
Phone: 609-452-0606 or 800-221-4792
Fax: 609-987-8116
Web: www.rfbd.org
E-mail: custserv@rfbd.org

Founded in 1948 to provide recorded textbooks to veterans blinded in World War II, RFB&D now makes educational material available at all academic levels in recorded and computerized forms for those,including dyslexics, unable to use standard print.

World Dyslexia Network Foundation
P.O. Box 3333
London SE21 8ZN
United Kingdom
Phone: 011-44-0181-761-7777
Fax: 011-44-0181-766-6281
Web: www.surrey.ac.uk/Psychology/WDNF

The WDNF was set up in 1995 "to serve the needs of the dyslexia community worldwide." It has a Web site with a variety of information and links, and helps produce the *International Book of Dyslexia.*

## Dyspraxia/Apraxia

American Speech-Language-Hearing Association
10801 Rockville Pike
Rockville, MD 20852
Phone: 301-897-5700 or 800-498-2071
Web: www.asha.org

This is an organization made up of speech language pathologists and audiologists, which also provides general information and referrals to the public with regard to speech, language, and hearing disorders.

Dyspraxia Foundation
8 West Alley
Hitchin
Herts SG5 1EG
United Kingdom

Phone: 011-44-1462-454986
Fax: 011-44-1462-455052
Web: www.emmbrook.demon.co.uk/dysprax/
    homepage.htm
The Dyspraxia Foundation supports individuals and families affected by developmental dyspraxia and aims to increase public understanding and awareness of the disorder. The organization issues a newsletter and its Web site has links to recent research and other sites. I have included this British organization because of the dearth of U.S. entities.

Madeleine Portwood
Web: http://web.ukonline.co.uk/members/madeleine.
    portwood/dysprax.htm
E-mail: madeleine.portwood@ukonline.co.uk
A specialist senior educational psychologist and author based in Durham, England, Madeleine Portwood is chairperson of the Education Committee of the Dyspraxia Foundation.

## General

All Kinds of Minds Institute
P.O. Box 3580
Chapel Hill, NC 27515
Phone: 919-933-8082
Fax: 919-967-3590
Web: www.allkindsofminds.org
All Kinds of Minds is a nonprofit institute that provides hands-on practical advice and tutoring to help children with learning difficulties. Founded and headed by Dr. Mel Levine, professor of pediatrics at the University of North Carolina Medical

School in Chapel Hill and director of the University's Clinical Center for the Study of Development and Learning.

American Academy of Child & Adolescent Psychiatry
3615 Wisconsin Avenue NW
Washington, DC 20016-3007
Phone: 202-966-7300
Fax: 202-966-2891
Web: www.aacap.org

This is the association of psychiatrists whose journal publishes many studies with regard to all aspects of ADHD. Through its Web site, the academy also provides information to aid in the understanding and treatment of developmental, behavioral, and mental disorders.

Center for Science in the Public Interest (CSPI)
1875 Connecticut Avenue NW, Suite 300
Washington, DC 20009
Phone: 202-332-9110
Fax: 202-265-4954
Web: www.cspinet.org
E-mail: cspi@cspinet.org

CSPI, founded in 1971, is a nonprofit health-advocacy organization that conducts research and advocacy programs in nutrition, food safety, and alcoholic problems. It is supported by the one million American and Canadian subscribers to its "Nutrition Action Healthletter" and by foundation grants.

The Council for Exceptional Children (CEC)
1920 Association Drive
Reston, VA 20191-1589
Phone: 703-620-3660 or 888-CEC-SPED

Fax: 703-264-9494
Web: www.cec.sped.org
E-mail: service@cec.sped.org
A nonprofit membership organization with seventeen
specialized divisions including the Division for Learning Disabilities, the Division for Children's Communication Development, and the Association for the Gifted. CEC and its divisions
hold conferences and publish newsletters and journals.

ERIC Clearinghouse on Disabilities and Gifted Education
    (ERIC EC)
The Council for Exceptional Children (CEC)
1920 Association Drive
Reston, VA 20191-1589
Phone: 800-328-0272
Web: http://eric.org
E-mail: ericec@cec.sped.org
ERIC is an acronym for the Educational Resources Informa-
tion Center. The ERIC Clearinghouse on Disabilities and Gifted
Education (ERIC EC) is one of sixteen nationwide information
networks sponsored by the U.S. Department of Education. The
database contains seventy thousand citations on disabilities or
gifted issues.

Council for Learning Disabilities
P.O. Box 40303
Overland Park, KS 66204-4303
Phone: 913-492-8755
Fax: 913-492-2546
Web: www.cldinternational.org
E-mail: webmaster@cldinternational.org
CLD is a national membership organization composed

of professionals who represent diverse disciplines and who are "committed to enhance the education and lifespan development of individuals with learning disabilities."

Learning Disabilities Association of America (LDA)
4156 Library Road
Pittsburgh, PA 15234-1349
Phone: 412-341-1515 or 888-300-6710
Fax: 412-344-0224
Web: www.ldanatl.org
E-mail: ldanatl@usaor.net
A nonprofit advocacy organization founded in 1964 by a group of concerned parents, LDA has over sixty thousand members with fifty state affiliates and is devoted to finding solutions for a variety of learning disorders. It provides information and referral services.

National Center for Learning Disabilities
381 Park Avenue South, Suite 1401
New York, NY 10016
Phone: 212-545-7510 or 1-888-575-7373
Fax: 212-545-9665
Web: www.ncld.org
E-mail: programs@ncld.org
A nonprofit organization, NCLD's mission is to promote public awareness and understanding of children and adults with learning disabilities. The organization provides information and educational tools for individuals with learning disabilities, parents, educators, and other professionals. It advocates for improved legislation and services for those with learning disorders.

National Information Center for Children and Youth with
    Disabilities (NICHCY)

P.O. Box 1492
Washington, DC 20013-1492
Phone: 202-884-8200 or 800-695-0285
Fax: 202-884-8441
Web: www.nichcy.org
E-mail: nichcy@aed.org

NICHCY is a national information and referral center that provides free information on disabilities and disability-related issues for families, educators, and other professionals. The Web site is a winner of the Health Improvement Institute's Aesculapius Award of Excellence for health-related Web sites.

National Institute of Child Health and Human
    Development (NICHD)
National Institutes of Health
Building 31, Room 2A32
Center Drive MSC 2425
Bethesda, MD 20892-2425
Phone: 301-496-5133
Fax: 301-496-7101

Provides reviews of literature and information for research conducted by the NICHD.

Schwab Foundation for Learning
1650 South Amphlett Boulevard, Suite 300
San Mateo, CA 94402-2508
Phone: 800-230-0988
Fax: 650-655-2411
Web: www.schwablearning.org
E-mail: infodesk@schwablearning.org

Founded in 1988 by discount brokerage pioneer Charles R. Schwab and his wife, Helen O'Neill Schwab, this organization is dedicated to raising awareness about learning differences and providing parents and teachers with the information, resources, and support they need to improve the lives of kids with such problems. The foundation's staff provides personal responses and customized information by phone and via the Internet.

Landmark College
RR1, Box 1000
River Road South
Putney, VT 05346
Phone: 802-387-6718
Web: www.landmarkcollege.org
Landmark is the only fully accredited college in the country designed exclusively for students with dyslexia, ADHD, and other learning disabilities. Located on a 125-acre campus in southeastern Vermont, it has a student/faculty ratio of three to one.

## Summer Camps

When you and your child both need a vacation why not send him or her to summer camp? There are camps around the country that specialize in taking care of children with learning disabilities. Here's how you can locate one that suits your needs.

American Camping Association (ACA), Inc.
5000 State Road 67 North
Martinsville, IN 46151-7902
Phone: 800-428-2267 or 765-342-8456
Web: http://www.acacamps.org
E-mail: customerservice@aca-camp.org
Their *Guide to ACA Accredited Camps* is free on the Web site. A printed copy is $14.95 (including shipping and handling).

Camp Channel, Inc.
Internet-only information
www.campchannel.com

Easter Seals—National Office
Easter Seals Camping and Recreation List
230 West Monroe Street, Suite 1800
Chicago, IL 60606
Phone: 800-221-6287 or 312-726-6200
Web: http://www.easter-seals.org
E-mail: nessinfo@seals.com

KidsCamps.com
5455 N. Federal Highway, Suite O
Boca Raton, FL 33487
Phone: 561-989-9330, Ext. 2
Fax: 561-989-9331
Web: www.kidscamps.com

Resources for Children with Special Needs
200 Park Avenue South, Suite 816
New York, NY 10003
Phone: 212-677-4650
Fax: 212-254-4070
Web: www.resourcesync.org
E-mail: resourcesnyc@prodigy.net
This nonprofit organization provides information and referrals, advocacy and training, and library services to New York City parents and caregivers of children with disabilities and special needs. Their special Camp Guide costs $24.50 including shipping and handling.

## SUMMER TREATMENT CAMPS

Summer Treatment Program (STP)
State University of New York at Buffalo
Department of Psychology
Park Hall
Buffalo, NY 14260
Phone: 716-645-3697
Web: http://wings.buffalo.edu/psychology/adhd

The STP is a clinical research program that offers state-of-the-art treatment to children with ADHD and related disorders. It is an intensive eight-week (Monday to Friday) day program that originated in 1980 and moved to Buffalo in 1996. Since 1993 it has been a core part of the major multisite Treatment Study for ADHD funded by the National Institute of Mental Health and the U.S. Office of Education. The same STP program was offered in the summer of 2000 at other sites including New York City; Nashville, Tennessee; Cleveland, Ohio; Johnstown, Butler, and Indiana, Pennsylvania; Charleston, South Carolina, and Ottawa, Canada.

# CHAPTER 12

# REAL-LIFE RESULTS

*If I can stop one heart from breaking,*
*I shall not live in vain;*
*If I can ease one life the aching,*
*Or cool one pain,*
*Or help one fainting robin*
*Unto his nest again,*
*I shall not live in vain.*

—EMILY DICKINSON

You're about to read what for some is the most important chapter in this book. So far you've heard about my family experience, which, combined with my nutritional background, led me to investigate more fully the connection between LCPs and learning disorders. You've read about ADHD, dyslexia, and dyspraxia and the biological basis of the genetic link between all three disorders. We've explored changes in the dietary and breast-feeding habits that have led to people in some developed countries today being deficient in these critical long-chain polyunsaturated fatty acids. I have described how you can put LCPs back into your diet (through supplementation and regular food), and I've suggested some "life skill" strategies for helping children with learning challenges. And, of course, of great importance is the latest groundbreaking scientific research demonstrating the merits of LCP supplementation.

Conducting scientific studies is an exciting yet often frustrating undertaking. It takes a long time to complete definitive research, and it can be very expensive. Quite frankly, I actually started to tell the story about how LCPs may help ADHD, dyslexia, and dyspraxia long before the definitive research was completed. Why did I do this? It is always difficult to know when you should start revealing potential benefits from nutritional intervention. In my long years as a nutritionist I have seen at least once how delay in changing common practice resulted in many more people suffering, and for longer than was necessary. Before it became public health policy, for instance, it had been well known for a long time that folic acid supplements would help prevent spina bifida.

With regard to our initial research, the results were pretty clear-cut even though there were so few people in the study. In this situation, the fact that small numbers were involved in the early clinical trials is of no real consequence. There weren't very many people, either, in the study in which James Lind discovered that lime juice cured scurvy. In fact, there were only two people in the group supplemented with lime juice. If a condition is closely related to a deficiency, small numbers can demonstrate efficacy. It is only when there is a rather tenuous link or small association between nutrition and a particular condition that you need large numbers to prove the link.

Of course, it is possible to have false positives with small numbers. That is why much more research was needed. However, as I was so aware of the challenges facing people with dyslexia and ADHD, I felt obliged to let these families know about the potential benefits as early as possible. The wide publicity following my first article on dyslexia and supplementation had definitely positive outcomes. Research on dyspraxia started much more quickly than would have happened otherwise. And as a direct result of that, many have now tried to good effect LCP supplements on related conditions such as apraxia. In all honesty, it really was not a difficult decision to make as it is widely recognized that, in any case, increased consumption of omega-3 fatty acids has health benefits for the population as a whole.

So why might this be the most important chapter in this book? Doctors prefer evidence-based medicine—double-blind, placebo-controlled clinical trials, in particular. And they are right to demand such rigorous testing before forming conclusive opinions. But we are dealing here with real people and real lives. From a parent's perspective it is almost as important to hear what has happened in the lives of others facing the same daily challenges. Over the last few years, I have received literally thousands of letters with questions from concerned parents and, I am delighted to say, numerous success stories. I'm sure you will be able to identify with some of the families to whom I would now like to introduce you—people who have already used LCP supplementation.

Some of the stories may sound incredible because the results have been so spectacular, but they are real people with real stories. I'd like to start with some dyslexia stories, because that's where I started, with my own family.

# DYSLEXIA

## Dramatic and Rapid Results

To my great delight I have been able to meet some of the enthusiastic parents who have written to me. Recently, on a visit to Australia, I met Ralph Morris, the father of nine-year-old Charlotte who suffers from dyslexia, although her main affliction is a very poor short-term memory. Ralph gave me the latest update on Charlotte's progress together with a delightful photograph of a beautiful girl with a beaming face. Originally, Ralph and his wife, Colette, had written me about Charlotte, saying, "Almost everything she learns is generally forgotten within the hour. This has made teaching very laborious and frustrating for all concerned—especially Charlotte." In desperation, over the years Ralph and Colette had tried various methods to help Charlotte, with only minor benefits.

A television documentary about LCP supplementation sparked their interest and, they say, within two weeks of using the Efalex supplement that was used in the clinical trials they began to see results. Wrote Ralph and Colette: "The improvements in Charlotte were so dramatic and rapid that if we had not seen them ourselves we would not have believed them. Two weeks after starting supplementation, Charlotte started reading signs from the back of the car and asking what they meant (exactly the same as one of the kids in the documentary). This was amazing, as Charlotte could not read anything unless she had memorized it. Also, she usually just sat in the back of the car and said nothing.

"We took her straight home and showed her a school spelling list of sixteen words (which she had not seen before). She wrote fifteen words correctly and made only one mistake. We corrected her on the mistake and asked her the next morning to write the sixteen words (by which time usually she would not have remembered *one* of the words). She got all sixteen words correct. Within five weeks of taking Efalex, Charlotte was reading simple books from cover to cover. By six weeks, Charlotte read her first Enid Blyton book (with a bit of difficulty with some words). Presently, Charlotte is reading books and text, which would have been impossible four months ago, even words she does not know. She is sounding them out and usually gets them (or close). She would not even have attempted this before."

Ralph and Colette went on to report that Charlotte had obtained 100 percent in her most recent class spelling review, that her mathematics had "improved significantly," and that she was attending a drama class and learning her script for an upcoming play. "But by far the major improvement has been in her self-esteem and motivation, both of which are sky high," they wrote. "Charlotte is no longer withdrawn and moody, and now believes she can catch up with the other kids in her class. She used to be a bit of an outcast at school, but now has a good number of friends and a great social life."

When I met Ralph, he told me that Charlotte had made phenomenal progress in artistic ability and craft skills and that she regularly wins prizes for her craftwork. In an exhibition in April 1999 she won a prize for the most outstanding work by a school student of any age.

## Christopher Catches Up

Back in the United Kingdom, one of the first families to write to me was Christine and Brian Marshall, who told me about their son, Christopher. In the beginning, Christine and Brian had just thought that their son was a bit slower than his brothers, Alistair and Duncan. But when he started school it became obvious that he was behind most of the other children in his class. After a couple of years at school, basic reading and spelling were still very difficult for him. He also found it hard to tie his shoelaces and do up buttons. And he was clumsy and uncoordinated. "He was pulling out his hair in clumps because of his frustration," recalls his mother. In fact, she says, he looked like an old-fashioned friar. Christopher's self-esteem and confidence plummeted. "He kept saying, 'I'm stupid.' He felt inferior," says Christine.

Christopher was officially identified as dyslexic at the age of eight after a full psychological assessment. Standardized reading, spelling, and comprehension tests showed that he was well behind his classmates. Although the diagnosis came as something of a relief, his progress was still very slow. Then Brian and Christine read about LCP supplementation in a national British newspaper and contacted me. Christine admits to initial skepticism. "I never thought it would work. It seemed such an unusual claim." After taking the supplement, Christopher became calmer and able to concentrate better, his hair started growing back, and he felt generally happier.

Within three months, Christopher's writing improved dramatically. "All these years we'd been waiting for him to write legibly. It seemed like three years' development happened in three months. I know it's not a cure but the worst of the symptoms are alleviated. Maybe those who take fatty acids now will stop dyslexia being passed on to the next generation," says his mother. After almost two years of LCP supplementation, Christopher's reading is standard for his age, and his spelling and comprehension have improved dramatically.

A dyslexia consultant who meets with Christopher on a weekly one-to-one session wrote to report: "Worthy of note is the fact that since taking part in the Efalex program, the level and length of time that Christopher is able to concentrate has improved. He is far less distractible or distracted by extraneous noise or movement. There are noticeable benefits for Christopher in taking this supplement. There has also been some improvement in the quantity and length of retention of concepts and amounts of information retained."

In addition, say Brian and Christine, "His confidence, happiness and health are without doubt much improved. He sleeps better, too. Christopher is a lovely boy with a real twinkle in his eye, but he is still overcoming the feelings of inadequacy, which his dyslexia has caused. It now looks like we are winning. Christopher himself has become much more positive."

The encouraging aspect of both of these stories about young dyslexics is the change from poor self-esteem and lack of ability to greater happiness and confidence. Often, when parents see such remarkable improvement, they are motivated to want to help other parents, too. Here are two such examples.

## Like Mother, Like Son

"I had learning problems as a child. My mother had learning problems. And I didn't want my child to suffer the same way." This is Wendy Stott of Rochester, Kent, in the United Kingdom talking about her son, Luke. Wendy first noticed that Luke had a problem when he was five years old. "He was very behind the other children and certainly behind his older brother. When you have your second child and he's not performing like the first, you think there must be something wrong," she says. "The teachers said he was just behind; that he was just slow. But frankly, they are not really trained to handle dyslexic children."

Wendy was concerned about Luke's overall aversion to reading and schoolwork. "He was not at all interested in books, like my other son. He found books boring. He was happy to sit in front of the TV all day. His language skills were not developing at all but he did like doing Legos. He hated play school—well, he liked the 'play' but not the 'school' part," she says. Wendy read about LCP supplementation in the publication *Dyslexia*. She began supplementing Luke with tablets, but after he had difficulty swallowing them switched to a liquid version.

Says Wendy: "It really seems to have improved Luke's memory and concentration. We notice when he's not taking it. He forgets things. You can't give him more than one instruction at a time. You might tell him to go upstairs for his sweater and shoes and when he gets there he can't remember what he's gone for. When he's not taking the supplement he's down and depressed. He seems much happier when he's taking it."

Wendy, who works as a classroom assistant in a state school, took a course in dyslexia so she could not only help Luke but also tutor other dyslexic children in the evenings. "I know a lot of other parents who gave supplements to their children and they've all been very pleased with the results," says Wendy. "It's very hard for someone who doesn't have a learning problem to understand what it's like. Some parents just don't understand and punish the child when it's not his fault. I like to try and help the children with the everyday running of their lives; getting organized, for example. Five minutes can seem like an hour to a dyslexic child!"

## Aiden Makes the Grade

Across the globe, in New Zealand, as early as the age of three, Aiden Silbery Shoji's parents could tell he was different from other children. There were specific problems. He had difficulty tying his shoelaces. He could not speak very well. And he was uncoordinated. On the other hand, he was obviously a bright child happy to spend long periods of time building complex Lego structures. He showed artistic promise, but while his drawings were highly detailed they were lacking in color.

By the second year of school, a negative comparison with his young peers was even more visible. His reading and handwriting skills were way behind the rest of the class. Unfortunately, an unenlightened teacher's response was to frequently slap Aiden with a ruler for "being naughty." The result: He became naughty, negative, and withdrawn. When he was seven, Aiden's mother, Angie, took matters into her own hands and contacted the Specific Learning Disabilities Association in Queensland, New Zealand, where he was assessed by a child psychologist. Usually unresponsive to "teacher types" or authority figures, Aiden reveled in the assessment process, which was conducted like a series of games.

Recalls Angie, "In all honesty, it was probably the most positive experience since he started school, showing him positive feedback on things he could do."

The psychologist's diagnosis was the turning point the family needed. He was at least of average intelligence, if not above. He was not dumb, just dyslexic. "Aiden cried and I did, too, but I was immediately sure we could work through it as a family," says Angie. "To me, his education began with that assessment. At last we knew that he was dyslexic and not slow as we had been told. We saw it as the ultimate challenge to see our son develop competency and rebuild his self-esteem."

The years since, of course, have not been easy, as Aiden's anxious parents tried to provide the best mix of support, encouragement, and discipline. A new school with an understanding headmaster made a big difference and Aiden's sporting talents were also encouraged. Further help came when Angie discovered LCP supplementation. Since taking supplements Aiden says that his powers of concentration have improved, he sleeps better, thinks he is less impulsive, and finds it much easier to study and focus at school. In the past he found it really hard to pay attention during the last period of the day, now he "hangs in there."

Aiden has now passed the School Certificate exam with high marks in English and is eagerly waiting the day he can go on to college. His remarkable progress has also been recognized and highlighted in other ways. He was selected as a member of the Queensland Youth Parliament, representing Print Disabled/Dyslexic Young People, and in May of 1998, the governor general, Sir Michael Hardy Boys, presented him with a Young Achievers Award in recognition of his outstanding accomplishments in his battle to overcome learning disabilities.

Today, Aiden is realistic about the challenges he faces. He says candidly, "You should try walking in my shoes. I have to think about my lessons a lot before I can convert it into knowledge.

Really, I have to try twice as hard as the other kids. It gets very tiring to be trying all the time and when I get low marks I get frustrated. But the good news is I am getting better and enjoy school more." Where does he go from here? Aiden is interested in psychology, would like to understand why he is dyslexic, and possibly work in the army as a psychologist. Angie has become so involved in the wider issues of learning disabilities that she is now the chief executive of the Specific Learning Disabilities Association.

These are some examples of how children with dyslexia have been helped. Children with ADHD, however, present a rather different array of problems for their parents. Not only do the parents have to contend with a constant whirlwind existence, but they are also offered a remedy in the form of stimulant medication. It is a decision that many are uncomfortable having to make. So, let's look at how some parents have been able to cope.

# ADHD

## Warning from the Womb

There were signs, even before he was born, that little Nick Eggers was going to be hyperactive. "He was very, very active in the womb," says his mother, Theresa. "He never stopped kicking and moving." Theresa was in labor for two days before a cesarean section finally brought Nick into the world. He continued being troublesome. "He never slept more than two hours at a time, and he wouldn't let me nurse him. For some reason he was much more happy with the bottle," says Theresa. At nursery school, she adds, "They just thought he was an undisciplined child, but I knew it wasn't a discipline problem. He was just active. I learned early on that he needed structure. Everything had to be done at the same time each day, which I had no problem doing because luckily I'm a stay-at-home mom."

Theresa put Nick into a private kindergarten and in a class of just ten children he received plenty of help from a young, enthusiastic teacher. But when he started first grade it was an entirely different story. He was hyperactive, always agitated. At the age of six, he was diagnosed with ADHD and his parents reluctantly decided to give him Ritalin. "I'd suspected that he had ADHD, but my husband, Bruce, didn't want to believe that," says Theresa. "After doing a lot of research, I showed it to Bruce and he finally accepted it. In fact, he also realized that he had ADHD himself. We could see it in his mother, too, and then he remembered that his grandmother was always hyper."

Feeling that the Ritalin was stunting Nick's growth and making him have no appetite, Theresa began to search for alternatives and over the next few years tried several different approaches without success. Then she ran into a nurse, whose son also had ADHD, who told her about LCP supplementation. At this time, says Theresa, in the evenings she could tell the minute Nick was coming off the Ritalin. "He would crash. He would get real agitated—not mean, because he's a tenderhearted kid, but he would cry and get very mad and upset. Nothing would satisfy him." In April of 1999, at the age of ten, Nick began to take an LCP supplement in addition to his morning and lunchtime doses of Ritalin. "The first thing I noticed was that he was beginning to eat a bit more and then he became much calmer in the evenings," says Theresa.

During the summer vacation, Theresa stopped giving the LCP supplement to Nick. There was plenty to keep him occupied on their forty-acre farm in Mount Pleasant, Michigan, and his behavior seemed fine. But not long after returning to school, his bad behavior prompted teachers to ask if he was still getting his Ritalin. "It wasn't until the teacher sent me a note saying, 'Are you sure you haven't changed his meds?' that it hit me," she remembers. The only difference was that he was not getting his LCP supplement. She immediately began giving it to him again and says that within days everyone could tell the difference: "It really levels him out. He doesn't get agitated in the evenings like he used to. He still finds it hard to concentrate on his homework. I have to be right there with him. But he's definitely a changed kid."

## "Go-go" Kyle Calms Down

Five-year-old Kyle Yellets is another whirlwind bundle of energy. "He has always been a 'go-go-go' kind of guy," says his mother, Domigene. But there had not been any out-of-control behavioral problems until the fall of 1998, when he started half day at a Christian kindergarten. "After about a week, the teacher told us that he was disrupting the class, that he was throwing tantrums and hitting and scratching the other kids," says Domigene, who was totally perplexed. "We could not believe it as we just didn't have these problems at home."

A couple of weeks later, his unruly behavior flared at home. "He began attacking us, too. He would hit, scratch, spit, and be disobedient. He was extremely defiant," remembers Domigene. "The tantrums were out-of-control episodes that lasted one to two hours. On the weekends he would have a couple of tantrums a day. We couldn't take him anywhere. One day we went to a Chinese restaurant because he said he wanted to eat there. When we got there he changed his mind and pitched a fit. I had to drag him onto the seat to get him to eat. But that was just typical of his behavior. He was very obstinate and very determined to get his own way."

Confesses Domigene, "It sounds awful, but we kind of let him make the decisions just so that he would behave. But as soon as we went along with something, he would change his mind. He would say he wanted spaghetti for dinner and when we sat down to eat, he didn't want it. It was constant. There was nothing you could do to soothe him or please him. Whenever we were in public and he was misbehaving, we heard all the classic comments. In the supermarkets and other places people would ask, 'Don't you discipline your child?' or 'Can't you make your child behave?' Even the pediatrician said that we should spank him more. We were already spanking him three or four times a day, and it wasn't doing any good."

Around Christmas 1998, Kyle was diagnosed as having ADHD and was prescribed Ritalin and Imipramine in the morning, and Imipramine in the evening. "This seemed to help him stay on task and he was getting his work done, but it did not help his behavior at all," says his mother. "He was still disrupting class and having the extreme temper tantrums, and he even cut a boy's shirt and a girl's hair. The teacher had to constantly keep moving him. Finally, she had a special chair right by her desk to segregate him from the other kids in the classroom. She thought he was going to seriously hurt the other children. He was spitting at them and scratching them. It was just a nightmare."

Domigene began to research ADHD, buying books on the subject and surfing the Internet. After reading about nutritional treatments including fatty acid supplementation, she began weaning Kyle off the Ritalin and onto the Efalex product, as well as trying to eliminate artificial dyes, flavors, preservatives, and trans fats from his diet.

Within two weeks, she says, they began to notice improvement. "He was definitely calmer and more compliant. He was able to express his anger verbally rather than wildly hitting and scratching." His temper tantrums, she says, decreased from as many as two or three a day to one a month—and they are the "normal" episodes one might expect from a five-year-old. They last fifteen to twenty minutes and Kyle doesn't hit anymore. "It's a night-and-day difference. He still gets upset, but no more than any five-year-old when he's tired. He's obedient. He actually tells me that he was wrong and I was right, something he would never do before." Domigene decided to test the effectiveness of Efalex by not obtaining anymore after her supply ran out. Result: "After a week he started throwing tantrums again!" she exclaims. Kyle is now back on two capsules in the morning and two at night.

## Stigma No More

In New South Wales, Australia, Michael and Karen Wicks are two other parents unhappy with the thought of stimulant medication. At age five, their son, Tyson, was diagnosed as having ADHD. Michael and Karen agreed with the diagnosis, but they did not agree quite so readily with the doctor's prescription: dextroamphetamine. "We were far from happy having our son taking amphetamines," they recall, "but after seeing the dramatic positive impact on his behavior we thought it was the best thing to do." The improvement in behavior, however, did not come without unpalatable side effects. "The dextroamphetamine produced a lack of appetite. We continually had to fight with Tyson to get him to eat. As a result, his growth slowed down."

Tyson's parents also noticed that he found it harder to control his behavior as the effect of one dosage diminished and it became time for the next to be administered. That, too, they saw as problematic. "He had to go to the school office every lunchtime to have the next tablet. This made him feel different. There must be a stigma with medication even at this age. Overall, the dex was working but it wasn't a happy situation." This lasted for two and a half years, until Michael and Karen came across LCP supplementation.

Initially, they substituted LCPs on weekends, discovering that "Saturdays were a bit erratic; Sundays were great. He was just like any other seven-year-old boy. Mondays at school were OK as well."

The results were so encouraging that Tyson's parents gave him a full-time trial on LCPs during the school holidays. When his behavior settled down after the first week and his behavior throughout the holidays was "as it should have been for a seven-year-old boy," they decided to permanently replace dextroamphetamine with LCPs. They say, "His appetite is normal. In fact, you have to tell him to stop eating. He has grown. He has gained weight and his behavior does not fluctuate as it did before."

## Life with Lucas

In Montreal, Canada, Alice Weiss says that the "terrible twos" hit with a vengeance—and didn't go away. At the age of two and a half, she says, her son Lucas became a little horror. "Everyone told me it was just the 'terrible twos' and I said, 'Oh, my God, they're more than terrible.' They said that it would change when he turned three. Finally, he became three and the terrible twos continued. Then he was four, and it wasn't getting any better. If anything, it was getting worse."

Alice recounts what life with Lucas was like: "He couldn't sit and watch TV. He couldn't sit and watch cartoons or a Disney movie. Nothing lasted for more than two minutes before he was on to the next thing. If you gave him crayons, after just a couple of minutes he'd throw them away laughing. Nothing held his attention except Legos. He'd do that for forty-five minutes. Everything else, he just broke. He could, however, construct the most incredible things. He would build these Lego things so tall and explain how they balanced. I could not make the things he was making at the age of three. It was unbelievable."

Lucas also had artistic talent. "His pictures would be very interesting. He wouldn't make a picture of a house, a person, and the sun, like a typical child. Everything was connected with lines and circles and stars. It was like his mind was going and going and like the picture was moving. He had thirty-six crayons and would use every color," says Alice. But Lucas's behavior imposed severe restrictions on their lifestyle. "I couldn't go anywhere. I couldn't take him to a shopping mall. If I did, I needed two other people to help monitor him. I'd tell him to hold my hand and before I knew it he'd dashed off somewhere. He was distracted in every single possible way. When we'd walk into a store he had to touch everything and he always had a million questions. I almost needed a tranquilizer just to go out with him."

At the age of four, Lucas began to demonstrate some extremely creative behavior at the dinner table. "He couldn't just sit in the chair," says Alice. "He would lie on his stomach, eating away on a piece of toast and moving his hands. It looked as if he was swimming! And forget restaurants. He would be sitting with everyone else in the restaurant except us. He would be in the kitchen to see what was going on, so I gave up on restaurants. It was exhausting, majorly exhausting."

When Lucas entered kindergarten, the teachers, suspecting ADHD, quickly recommended a psychiatric evaluation. "They said he showed all the signs of ADHD and suggested Ritalin, but they didn't know for sure," remembers Alice. "I said, 'I'm not putting him on Ritalin when you're telling me you're not 100 percent sure. Would you put someone on heart medication if you weren't sure they had a heart condition?' " Lucas was barely five years old. Every few days there were notes from school. "I would get these notices saying, Lucas did this or Lucas did that. He took the scissors and cut the glue stick instead of doing his work. He was looking out of the window instead of listening to the story. He was always touching the kids sitting in front of him. He could never leave them alone. They had different workstations in the classroom but he could never finish a task at one before it was time to move on to the next."

Close to the end of his kindergarten year, everyone began wondering what would happen to Lucas in first grade, because he simply couldn't sit still in a chair. A special program was suggested—a small class of just eight children, with a teacher and psychologist. Around this time Alice picked up a magazine, read about LCP supplementation, and decided to try it.

At first, Lucas had difficulty swallowing the capsules and disliked the taste. Says Alice: "I told him to keep trying as it would make him feel better. I wasted quite a few, but he kept saying, 'I'm going to do it. I'm going to do it.' One day, after three weeks, he managed it without a problem. Now he can swallow four at a time, washed down with water!" It was two months before Alice started noticing changes. "He wasn't this wild, crazy child anymore. There were still some issues to deal with, such as impulsivity, but he could sit in a chair like a person, instead of like a fish. He would sit and read a book with me without his legs going all over the place. Before supplementation, when he was reading to me, he would often get to the end of a line and completely skip the next line or start reading in the middle of the next line. After supplementation, he could read properly and pronounce words he couldn't pronounce before. He's not as wound up. He's able to concentrate better. And his behavior is so much improved that we can actually take him to restaurants."

There have also been improvements at school. Says Alice: "He's in a regular class and on his report card he got a 'satisfactory.' That's unbelievable considering where he was coming from. He even got an A for penmanship, and his writing used to be atrocious. He would write one big letter, then one small letter, and the next letter almost sideways. His writing now looks like that of a ten-year-old. It used to take him an hour to do five minutes' work. Now it's a breeze.

I forgot to give him the supplement one week and I realized what had happened when I saw his writing going backwards again."

Some of the most dramatic breakthroughs, however, have been reported by parents of children with dyspraxia, and particularly apraxia of speech. As no research studies have yet been conducted with apraxic children, these accounts are the only evidence we have. The following is just a selection. Many more parents have described and discussed their experiences with us and on the Internet.

# Dyspraxia/Apraxia

## The "Lellow" Breakthrough

Three-year-old Tanner, standing in the bathroom of his family's New Jersey home, picked up a pink comb, pointed to a yellow stripe that ran through it, and said, "Lellow." It was the first "real" word he had ever spoken and it came after just three weeks of supplementation. "I almost fell over," says his delighted mother, Lisa Geng. "It was the breakthrough we had been waiting for. It was incredible." Within a few days, Tanner's vocabulary increased to seven words. Within five weeks, he had mastered twenty-two words.

During his first year of life, Tanner had seemed like a normal, healthy baby, and by the age of eleven months was babbling normally and saying "ma" and "da." Then, after a bout of very high fever, he stopped talking. Photographs show an unsmiling two-year-old. "No matter how hard the photographers tried he just would not smile. He was lethargic," says Lisa. Typically, everyone kept telling her that he was just a late talker, but Lisa and her family became increasingly concerned and pushed for a hearing and speech evaluation. Four months of speech therapy led to an official diagnosis of severe apraxia. Tanner was two years, eight months old. During the four months of speech therapy he had learned to say basic sounds such as *sh*, *ch*, *t*, and *s* with some prompting. He had learned how to blow bubbles and could move his mouth more than before. But he found it impossible to take the *ch* sound and put it together with the *oo* sound to make "choo."

As soon as they heard that Tanner was apraxic, Lisa and her husband, Glenn, began to search for information. "We were shocked to find out how little support and information there was at the local level, and this was in a fairly affluent area close to New York," says Lisa. In desperation, the couple turned to the Internet and discovered the apraxia-kids listserv. After reading other parents' positive comments about LCP supplementation and consulting Lisa's aunt, a retired nursing teacher at Long Island University, they decided to give it a try.

Three weeks later they were thrilled with the results of that decision. "I know that it can take as long as three months of supplementation for any benefits to be noticed, but we saw results with Tanner in three weeks. I'm not exaggerating," says Lisa. Tanner's Early Intervention therapist told them that he had become "a different child" and the therapist was so impressed that she began recommending LCP supplementation to other patients.

Lisa and Glenn, however, took him off supplementation for a while when he was going through testing for the disabled preschool program in their hometown. "His improvement had been so dramatic we were actually afraid that he would test too well to be accepted," says Lisa. The result was calamitous. "It was the saddest thing. We will never do that to him again. The poor little thing was no longer able to say as much, and he just didn't seem to learn. He wasn't able to 'parrot' us like he had when taking the supplements. And for the first time he was frustrated to the point of tears."

Back on supplementation, Tanner showed steady improvement and broadened his vocabulary. Adds Lisa: "He's able to say many things now. Just last night he looked at his daddy, and said, 'Love you.' What a wonderful moment that was." Lisa says that the only negative is trying to get Tanner to actually take the supplements, because of the fishy taste. She does her best to disguise it by mixing the contents of the capsules with cereal and other foods.

Lisa and Glenn became so interested in helping Tanner and other kids like him that they started a nonprofit organization, Children's Apraxia Network, based at the Children's Specialized Hospital in Mountainside, New Jersey. One of the group's main goals is to raise funds to enable parents of "late-talking children" to have consultations with speech language pathologists when their kids are at an earlier age. Says Lisa: "What parents hear is, 'Wait until he's three and then we'll run some tests.' That's too late when a child has a real problem and should be getting treatment earlier."

## Kelli's Three-Syllable Breakthrough

On the West Coast, in San Jose, California, little Kelli Sheehy, at the age of four, only had a vocabulary of about one hundred, single-syllable words. Rarely could she manage to say two consecutive syllables with correct pronunciation in the correct order. Her motor skills were also cause for concern. She could not balance well enough to walk up stairs or jump off a curb. She was still not potty trained. Her family was really discouraged. In spite of all their efforts and regular speech therapy, Kelli's progress was excruciatingly slow.

Kelli's mother, Kathie Sheehy, had first noticed that something was wrong when Kelli was one year old. "She wasn't speaking as much as her two older siblings had done at the same age. I mentioned it to the pediatrician and he said it wasn't a problem and to wait until her eighteen-month checkup. She was no better then, but he said she was within norms and to wait until she was two and a half. As soon as she hit that age I insisted that there had to be a problem and that I needed a referral to a speech therapist."

The pediatrician agreed and the speech therapist identified apraxia. Kelli began therapy and Kathie found a school for her that was "speech language intensive." Progress was slow. After six to eight months, Kelli was able to pronounce some two-syllable words. "Nevertheless it was an accomplishment," says Kathie. "Before she went to the speech therapist she only had the ability to say about two one-syllable words and some words of two repetitive syllables. She would say 'ba-ba' for 'bottle' and 'mamma' was anyone in authority who could help her, like mom, dad, and big sister."

The prognosis was that Kelli would be speaking understandably by the age of six or seven through intensive speech therapy. But Kathie wanted more for her child. She turned to the Internet, found the apraxia-kids list and the discussion about the benefits of LCP supplementation. "I couldn't see anything in the ingredients that would hurt my daughter and decided to go with it," she says.

Within six weeks, she began to see "dramatic improvements" both in Kelli's communication and gross motor abilities, epitomized by an event one morning that she'll never forget. "I was reading her the *101 Dalmatians* book," says Kathie. "I pointed to the picture of one of the young dogs, and asked her to tell me what it was. I expected Kelli to say 'dog,' and would have been extremely pleased to hear her say 'puppy.' Instead, she responded 'Dalmatian' with perfect articulation. This amazed me because up until then she had never uttered any word without weeks of practice, much less a three-syllable word. And because of turnover at her communication school, Kelli had not had any speech therapy with a good SLP [speech language pathologist] for the previous three weeks. I had no reason to expect any progress, much less advancement of this magnitude."

The next week, Kelli amazed her mother even more. She began to sing the "Alphabet Song" with stunningly correct sequencing and articulation, including the ending sentences, "Now I've sung my A-B-C's, Next time won't you sing with me?" Adds Kathie: "I was astounded at her ability to remember so many words in the correct order since no one was practicing these skills with her at that time. It was like someone had put a key in the lock and opened the door wide open. Soon afterward we had a chance to see the teacher from the speech intensive school, who hadn't seen Kelli for eighteen months, and she was just blown away." Kelli's motor skills also began to improve. Potty training took less than two weeks, with few accidents, says Kathie. And Kelli began maneuvering up and down stairs with ease and even began to ride a bicycle with training wheels.

Today, Kelli is doing well in a regular first-grade classroom. She now speaks with 98 percent understandability, although she still has some difficulty sequencing words and describing things. Says her mother: "The bottom line is that she's reading six months ahead of her level instead of being two years behind, as predicted. The teachers are amazed at her writing ability both in copying words and coming up with her own. Her spelling is age-appropriate, but the teacher is incredibly impressed with her thoughts and the way that she is expressing herself. She has such a creative mind. We were so surprised and thrilled because we were prepared for her not to be in a normal classroom, much less reading above average."

## Clearing Away the Fog

"Any day now. Don't worry. It will come. Any day now and he'll start talking." All year long, Conrad's speech therapist had kept reassuring his parents that it was just a matter of time before their only child would break his silence. Alarmed at his inability to speak by his second birthday, they had taken him to the therapist. But now, Conrad was almost three years old and still couldn't speak a word. "That's when I decided it was time to take charge," says his mother, Janice Goldschmidt.

She took Conrad to a pediatric neurological specialist who diagnosed his problem as severe apraxia. "It was a brutal diagnosis," says Janice, "but at least we knew exactly what we were dealing with." As far as his parents were concerned that meant launching their own campaign to do everything they could to help him achieve his full potential. They located excellent speech therapists, organized one-on-one treatment, and personally, painstakingly threw themselves into a daily program of oral motor exercises.

In addition to the physical therapy, his parents began to investigate nutritional treatment and heard about LCP supplementation. "I was skeptical at first, but I consulted a nutritionist and she said it was nothing that could hurt him, so we decided to give it a try." The Goldschmidts of Arlington, Virginia, began to give their son 240 milligrams of DHA a day. Within six weeks, Conrad had learned three new consonants. That doesn't sound too impressive, until you consider that he'd learned just one consonant in the previous two months.

After twelve weeks they were happy to report marked improvement. "The supplement is clearly helping him. It's as if it has cleared up some fog inside his head. There's a 10 to 20 percent improvement, and in the world of apraxia that is huge," says his mother. Adds Janice: "Every week now, Conrad experiments with new sounds and vowel combinations. Speech therapy is extremely important, but I wouldn't dream of taking him off the supplement because I've seen what it has done for him." Conrad is basically "very smart," says his mother. He has "a huge desire" to talk and learn and has an extensive "receptive" vocabulary, understanding much of what is said to him. But he is also behind other children of his age in the development of his handwriting, gross motor ability ("a little bit clumsy"), and his ability to mix with other children.

One year after the initial diagnosis of apraxia, Janice says, "Every week there is a little progress. Every week there's an improvement in his speech." Conrad can count to ten, can "make things equal" up to eight, and has been learning appropriate use of pronouns. His kindergarten teacher says that he has become much more able to follow directed play. Says Janice: "My job is to get my son ready for school and I'm going to do it. It's my job. He's not going into special ed!"

Interestingly, like many families with learning disorders, Conrad's challenges spurred family reflections on the issue and the revelation that at the age of three his grandfather had been placed in a special program for speech delay and had had a stuttering problem. A modern diagnosis would almost certainly say that he had had apraxia, says Janice.

## Unlocking Seth's Voice

At the age of three, little Seth Kvam had very few "real" words in his vocabulary. He did, however, have a language of his very own. For instance, he called his mother "Aw-bee." His sister, Kristy, was "I-ya," dogs were "babas," cats were "ryes," and juice was "ju." In total, there were about twenty made-up words that Seth consistently used. "He made them up and we learned them," says his mother, Paula Kvam. "His sister, who's three years older, was a wonderful interpreter. They're very close and she always knew what he was saying. Seth would also point at things and pretty much get his message across."

At his three-year checkup, Seth's pediatrician had expressed concern about his inability to talk and insisted on an evaluation.

Paula and her husband were reluctant. "I think we were in denial," she says. "We just wanted to believe everyone who was saying that he would catch up." Seth entered special ed preschool through his local school district in Camano Island, Washington, and began receiving speech therapy. He improved a little, but with kindergarten just a year away Seth's therapist was concerned because he was still so far behind. "He would confuse pairs of sounds like *p* and *b*. It was really hard to understand him," says Paula.

In February 1999, in addition to school therapy, Seth began to receive private therapy, but by and large could not be understood by anyone outside his immediate family. In April, Paula got on the apraxia-kids listserv and began reading all about LCPs. On May 25 she began giving him an LCP supplement every day (along with a Gummi bear to mask the taste). "Within three weeks his voice was unlocked," says Paula. "Within a month his intelligibility increased from 40 to 50 percent to 85 to 90 percent and he is still improving."

On July 23, 1999, Seth's private therapist verified his improvement using the Goldman-Fristoe Test of Articulation. He reported that all speech sounds within the five-and-a-half-year developmental level were being correctly produced. Perhaps most astonishing of all: All of Seth's gains came when he was not getting any speech therapy and no speech practice at home, either.

Says Paula: "The change in Seth has been amazing. He is now a normal little boy. He still has a few speech errors, but he can say just about anything and everything. He is understood almost all of the time by others and he can communicate freely with us. He has so much fun playing with all the other little boys. He's right in the middle of it. He's always been a happy kid. He was never angry or frustrated at his inability to communicate because his sister could always interpret for him. It was as if they had their own secret language. But now a whole new world's opened up for him."

According to Seth's speech therapist, in just four months the youngster went from being "largely unintelligible" to "highly intelligible." In a report, the therapist wrote that in May 1999 his speech was "largely unintelligible to unfamiliar listeners. At that time Seth's parents began supplementing his diet with fatty acids after reading anecdotal data on the topic. By September 1999, Seth's oral motor planning and sequencing skill had improved substantially and he had become highly intelligible during conversational speech." After four months of supplementation, the six-year-old boy who could barely talk was now testing at the level of an eight-year-old.

## Cody, Cameron, and Cory

Like the children you've met already—Tanner, Kelli, Conrad, and Seth—young Cody Hartley basically couldn't talk. His mother, Valerie Hartley, had been concerned for quite a while, but the experts had constantly reassured her that "he was just delayed." Concern quickly escalated into alarm when Cody's brother, Cameron, fifteen months his junior, passed him by, and began to develop an ever-expanding vocabulary. "That's when I said, 'Something is not right. This is more than just a delay,'" remembers Valerie, who lives near Erie, Pennsylvania. It had been obvious to Valerie that Cody's development had been slower than that of his older brother, Cory. "But everybody told me that the second child was often slower," she says. "They said that the first child did the talking for the second, but I knew that wasn't the case. My son was basically unintelligible. I couldn't understand him. It was bad. Life was miserable for him and the rest of us. The poor kid couldn't get across to his mother what he wanted. He might want to have some juice, but couldn't communicate what he needed. He would get mad, and throw temper tantrums. I would get mad, and feel terrible. He would cry and I would cry."

Beginning to fear that Cody would never lead a normal life, Valerie quit her job as a certified public accountant so that she could devote more time to helping him. At the same time Valerie and husband, Dan, invested in twice-weekly private speech therapy sessions. The $350-a-month cost was coming out of their own pockets because insurance would not cover the treatment. They saw some improvement during the first six months, and then nothing more.

With the family budget in jeopardy she pulled him from the private therapy in January of 1999 and desperately began to look for help elsewhere. Closely reading a report from the speech therapist she came across the term "apraxia of speech." Valerie turned to the Internet to find out more. "It opened a whole new world for me," she says. "Within a week I had a twelve-page report on the subject and I said, 'This is Cody. This is what Cody is.' " A neurologist and another speech pathologist subsequently agreed. Further research on the Internet led to the apraxia-kids listserv and the discovery that a group of parents were enthusiastically discussing the benefits of LCP supplementation. She decided to give it a try. No one other than Valerie and Dan knew. "The results were incredible!" exclaims Valerie. "Within a month his teachers were telling me how they were starting to understand him. They thought the speech therapy was helping him, but at this stage he wasn't having any speech therapy. The only thing different was the LCP supplementation."

One year after starting supplementation, Valerie says Cody's progress has been "amazing," adding, "He talks with 90 percent intelligibility. He does leave the endings off words and sometimes talks fast and I have to get him to slow down. But most of the time I know what he's talking about and he's a much happier little boy. No temper tantrums, that's for sure. He does talk mostly in sentences, but often leaves out words like 'the' and 'this.' If he's in a hurry, it's as if he resorts almost to telegraphic speech using just the most important words."

Cody is now six years old and in kindergarten. His teacher understands him most of the time and when the teacher doesn't the other kids do, yelling out a word that Cody has said so that the teacher can get it. A speech therapist, who tested Cody in February 1999 and again in June "couldn't believe the difference," says Valerie.

As I've explained elsewhere in this book, it is quite common for children to suffer from a combination of learning disorders. Here are just a few examples: a young boy with ADHD-Inattentive type combined with dyspraxia; another youngster who appeared to have both dyslexia and dyspraxia; and a third with dyspraxia and apraxia of speech.

## COMBINED DISORDERS

### Fast Brain, Slow Hands

Young Shane Collins of Granite Falls, Washington, has the inattentive form of ADHD, but that's not all. "We should have called him 'Pig Pen.' That would have been an appropriate nickname," says his mother, Melissa. "He was so untidy and disorganized. His bedroom and desk areas were utter disaster. His clothes and even his treasures, his sports trophies and cards, were strewn all over the place. He could lay his hands on whatever he wanted, but to everyone else it was just a terrible mess."

Untidiness wasn't Shane's only problem. Diagnosed with ADHD while in first grade, he was constantly fidgety and had concentration and focus problems. "He wasn't hyperactive at all. He did not have any wild, unruly behavior—quite the opposite, he has always been extremely well-behaved and eager to please," says Melissa. "But even if he could concentrate during a particular day, he had great difficulties keeping up with the rest of the class when doing tasks such as copying from the board. His brain could think much faster than his hands could write. He would get frustrated and feel totally lost and left behind."

Shane's problem only came to light when he started school. He had difficulty paying attention and was obviously not following instructions as well as his classmates. The class sizes were small and the teachers gave him as much individual attention as they could. Shane also displayed symptoms—not diagnosed—of dyspraxia. "He did not run and move like the other children. He has always been large for his age and was always clumsy and uncoordinated. He's very bright and was well aware that he moved differently than the other kids and he was becoming very self-conscious about it," says his mother.

Later, at a different school with larger classes and a not-so-understanding teacher, life became very difficult for Shane. "The attitude was just horrible," says Melissa. When he was in the fifth grade, the school wanted to put him on Ritalin and she refused. It was reminiscent of Melissa's own childhood. "I was diagnosed as hyperactive when I was about six years old and put on Ritalin for a while, but when my mother saw what it was doing to me she stopped it. Apparently I was calmer but spacey and just not myself. Instead, my mother decided to just cope with me. She didn't want me on drugs." Melissa took the same approach with her own child. She decided to home-school while searching for a natural alternative.

Melissa surfed the Internet for two years. It was a search that ended only when she came across a site discussing the merits of fatty acid supplementation in general and Efalex in particular that had enough evidence to satisfy her. As a result, she began to supplement Shane with LCPs. "We have had tremendous results. Shane, himself, even said to me that he found he was concentrating better. I can now understand his handwriting. It is much clearer, and it wasn't long ago that it was worse than that of his sister, who's five years younger. He is much more confident. He is an intelligent boy and he was well aware that he was not performing to the best of his ability and was somewhat different from the other kids," says Melissa. "He's now succeeding in his studies and *on his own* has organized all of his schoolbooks. He's categorized and filed away his work, and he designs his own daily routine. It's absolutely unbelievable. He's gone up at least one grade level in math, which is his most difficult subject. And on the Children's Skills Test, Self-Assessment software that I have he scores a grade equivalent of 11.7 in science."

Melissa is quick to add, "Don't get me wrong, he still has bad days, but what child doesn't? But he is not nearly as jumpy, twitchy, or 'drifty' as he used to be. His mind still works quickly and if his interests are fed and encouraged, he excels." Shane is now thirteen years old, five feet ten inches tall, and is becoming an adept athlete. "After six months of taking the supplements he is moving much more gracefully and with more control and confidence. He also doesn't struggle as much with tasks requiring fine movements and lots of hand-eye coordination. In fact, this is the first year that he has asked for model cars and is enjoying them. We got him one in the past and he was so frustrated with it, he threw it out."

Shane's skin is not so dry, his hair is silkier, and he has fewer allergy problems. He doesn't get the severe hay fever he used to. He doesn't have the frequent thirst and urination. "Until I began to research the subject I had no idea these were classic symptoms of fatty acid deficiency," says Melissa. Shane's younger brother, six-year-old Adam, displayed signs of hyperactivity as well, and since being supplemented has also become calmer and more in control. Other symptoms such as dry skin, eczema, and of course, dry hair have improved, too.

Melissa decided to take the supplement along with her children "so they wouldn't feel alone" and has also experienced benefits. "I can think more clearly and I have a more constant energy level." But the first change was physical. "For more than ten years I'd suffered with eczema on my right hand after working with chemicals. It disappeared in six to eight weeks."

## The King Midas Revelation

Over in the United Kingdom, meanwhile, five-year-old Alex Berridge was struggling to read. "It would take him a long time," says his mother, Pam Berridge. "He would get a word on one page but wouldn't recognize it on the next. He was also very slow at writing things down, especially when it meant copying them from the blackboard."

For the next few years progress continued to be slow with the teachers saying that he was "just behind" and "just being Alex." One day, just how far behind he really was hit home to Pam. Alex's homework assignment was to write the story of King Midas and the Minotaur. Says Pam, head of radiography at Cranfield University in Bedfordshire: "He was perfectly capable of telling me the story in graphic detail, but he wasn't capable of writing it down. The only way I could get him to write it down was for him to tell it to me a sentence at a time and for me to repeat it back to him one word at a time. And even then he was spelling it all wrong. It really rattled me."

Help came in the form of an educational psychologist who was working with some of Pam's university students. After hearing of Alex's problems the psychologist suggested an informal meeting before doing a full assessment. The outcome: At the age of eight and a half, Alex had a reading age of eight, a spelling age of seven, and an IQ of 142. A year later he was getting extra schooling through the Dyslexia Institute. At the age of nine and a half, he had a reading age of ten, but his spelling age was only seven years, three months.

Around the same time Alex was also diagnosed as dyspraxic. He was very tall for his age, and clumsy. He was uncoordinated and not very good at sports. He couldn't catch a ball. He was also fidgety, had an extremely short concentration span, and had difficulty tying his shoelaces. "But the main thing that screamed at us was his problems with writing. Even at the age of ten and a half he was still not writing automatically," says Pam. "He was having to tell his hand to go up and down and go round, as well as having to remember what letter, in what word, in what sentence, and how to spell it. Asking him to write his name was like asking him to climb Mount Everest. The very fact that he was coping all right at school just goes to show how determined he was and what a hard worker he was. The amount of effort he must have been putting in was phenomenal."

Luckily, Alex's grandmother read about LCP supplementation in a newsletter and Pam got in touch with me. After we discussed their situation, she decided to begin supplementing Alex. The first noticeable difference happened unusually quickly. Says Pam: "Alex was always very slow getting dressed in the mornings. He would daydream a lot. I would go into his room and he would be sitting there with just one sock on gazing out the window. One particular morning we overslept. I shot out of bed and ran into Alex's room, shouting, 'Come on. We're late. You've got to get up.' A few minutes later I went back to say, 'I mean it. You have to get up.' And he walked out fully dressed. My jaw just about hit the floor. I couldn't believe it."

As time went by the teachers began to notice a difference. It wasn't dramatic, but they said that he was concentrating better and was more focused. He'd begun to play tennis to try and help his dyspraxia, and the coach said that he was focusing better on the tennis court, and for longer periods of time. Previously, after hitting a few balls, he would be watching the birds! At Pam's university, one of her students, a twenty-six-year-old dyslexic male, also began taking LCP supplements. "Instead of getting up from his computer every five minutes to make a cup of coffee, or whatever, he found he could sit and concentrate for long periods. It made a profound difference. When he stopped taking the Efalex he reverted back to his restlessness. When he went back on the supplement his concentration came back," says Pam.

Recently, because of his learning challenges, eleven-year-old Alex was granted extra time to take exams. The teacher predicted he would get a grade three. Grade four is average for an eleven-year-old. "Well, Alex didn't need the extra time and he got grade five, an average for a thirteen-year-old," says Pam, proudly, adding, "Alex is a highly intelligent and popular child but his hesitancy and frustration with writing was a great stumbling block. His schoolwork is now definitely much improved, and while he has always been extremely competent, his work is now drawing praise from his teachers."

## "My Mouth Won't Talk"

Little Ryan Walden knew what he wanted to say but the words just wouldn't come out. He couldn't even say his own name or "mummy" and "daddy." Tripping over his tongue was only part of it. Physically uncoordinated, he seemed to trip over anything in his path. He couldn't figure out how to maneuver his legs to ride his bicycle. Frustrated beyond belief he resorted to temper tantrums. This was Ryan at the age of four—before his mother discovered LCPs.

Ryan's mother, Stacey Walden, had first noticed that her son was different when he was about fourteen months old. She worked at the preschool he attended and became painfully aware that other children who had been born around the same time were happily talking, but Ryan could barely mutter a few words. Says

Stacey: "I was really worried, but everyone said, 'He's a boy. He's the second child. Don't be worried. He'll talk when he's ready.' " But Stacey was also concerned because Ryan was behaving strangely. Close to the age of two, he played by himself all the time rather than with other kids. As he got older it became apparent that he hated groups of people. "At Thanksgiving and Christmas he was terrible around people. He was obviously uncomfortable. He would wring his hands and leave the room. He was having a lot of tantrums. They weren't triggered by anything I could pinpoint. Nothing in particular would seem to set him off," says Stacey.

Ryan was put into an Early Intervention program, but they kept telling his mother that he was "just delayed." The speech therapy, says Stacey, didn't seem to be helping, but the therapist kept saying he would "catch up." When Ryan was four, a new speech therapist recommended a comprehensive evaluation at the local hospital and Ryan was officially diagnosed as apraxic. It was July 1999. "It was a relief in many ways to have a name for it, to know what we were looking at," says Stacey in the family home near Iowa City, Iowa.

Like many other mothers, now that she knew her son had a specific problem, Stacey embarked on a mission to learn more. On the Internet, she found the apraxia-kids listserv. "There was a lot of discussion about fatty acids, a lot of people were saying how supplementation had done wonders for children with apraxia of speech," she remembers. "So I asked the pediatrician about it and he said it couldn't do any harm to try." Within two weeks of Ryan starting LCP supplementation, says Stacey, he was definitely trying to communicate with the spoken word more than through pointing and gesturing. The first big breakthrough, though, came in another way. Ryan had also displayed many symptoms of dyspraxia—poor motor coordination and general clumsiness. He had a bicycle but never rode it without the help of his parents pushing him down the street.

"I really knew the supplement was working when the child voluntarily hopped on his bike and pedaled away down the street by himself, while my husband and I stared with our jaws dropped. We were thrilled when he just took off by himself," says Stacey. As far as Ryan's speech was concerned, Stacey says that prior to supplementation, his vocabulary was extremely limited. "He used a few sounds to mean almost everything. He would use the word 'boo' for 'shoe,' 'juice,' and 'pooh.' He could say many words during his speech sessions, but did not retain them afterward. He left consonants off words, would shorten words down to one syllable, and leave the ends off words. Now, six months later, Ryan is speaking in sentences."

Says Stacey: "He can hold conversations with strangers, and they can understand most of what he says. He still has a long way to go before being completely intelligible, but he is definitely on his way. He has made more improvements in the six months of using the supplement than he had in the two years prior with speech therapy. Six months ago he could speak ten to twelve words clearly. Now he can say more than two hundred clearly and a lot of others not so clearly."

Adds Stacey: "When he was two he had said a few words such as 'hot,' 'bye bye,' and 'pizza.' He could say 'peek' (but not 'peek-a-boo') and he could say his own name, but then it was lost to him. He couldn't really even say mommy and daddy. That's only happened this year at the age of four. That only came back to him this year. Ryan's behavior has also improved. His tantrums have lessened. He's calmed down a lot now. His teachers and school speech therapist were stunned at how much he had progressed over the summer."

## Back to the Beginning—James's Story

The touchstone for my research, as you read in the introduction to this book, was the discovery that my son, James, had dyslexia. You may be wondering what happened to him. I'm pleased to tell you that the combination of LCP supplementation and tutor support helped him enormously. He made fantastic progress in spelling and other language skills. He actually won a place in one of the most competitive-entry academic schools in the United Kingdom. And won the "progress prize" in his first year.

James is now fifteen years old and has been taking an LCP supplement for five years. He is not very impaired by his dyslexia, but some characteristic traits remain. He still prefers to talk rather than write, for example. James probably wishes his mother would stop talking about him, although he hasn't complained. He recognizes his own strengths and weaknesses, and proudly wears the T-shirt of the SPELD organization of Australia with the logo: "Dyslexics of the World Untie."

# BIBLIOGRAPHY

## BOOKS

Amen, Daniel G., M.D. *Windows into the A.D.D. Mind. Understanding and Treating Attention Deficit Disorders in the Everyday Lives of Children, Adolescents and Adults.* Fairfield, Calif.: MindWorks Press, 1997.

American Psychiatric Association. *Diagnostic and Statistical Manual of Mental Disorders, 4th ed. (DSM-IV).* Washington, D.C.: American Psychiatric Association, 1994.

*Attention Deficit Hyperactivity Disorder.* National Health and Medical Research Council. Canberra, Australia: 1996.

Ayres, A. Jean. "Developmental dyspraxia and adult onset apraxia." Torrance, Calif.: Sensory Integration International, 1985.

Barkley, Russell A. *Attention-Deficit Hyperactivity Disorder. A Handbook for Diagnosis and Treatment.* New York: Guilford Press, 1990.

———. *Taking Charge of ADHD—The Complete, Authoritative Guide for Parents.* New York: Guilford Press, 1995.

Baumer, Bernice H. *How to Teach Your Dyslexic Child to Read: A*

*Proven Method for Parents and Teachers.* New York: Birch Lane Press, 1996.

Boyles, Nancy S., M.Ed, and Darlene Contadino, L.S.W. *Parenting a Child with Attention Deficit/Hyperactivity Disorder.* Los Angeles: Lowell House, 1996.

Breggin, Peter R., M.D. *Talking Back to Ritalin: What Doctors Aren't Telling You About Stimulants for Children.* Monroe, Maine: Common Courage Press, 1998.

Brown, Mick. *Richard Branson. The Authorized Biography.* London: Headline Book Publishing, 1998.

Carlson, Trudy. *Learning Disabilities. How to Recognize and Manage Learning and Behavioral Problems in Children.* Duluth, Minn.: Benline Press, 1997.

Carper, Jean. *Your Miracle Brain.* New York: HarperCollins, 2000.

Cherkes-Julkowski, Miriam; Susan Sharp; and Jonathan Stolzenberg. *Rethinking Attention Deficit Disorders.* Cambridge, Mass.: Brookline Books, 1997.

Cocks, Neralie. *Watch Me, I Can Do It! Helping Children Overcome Clumsy and Uncoordinated Motor Skills.* East Roseville, NSW, Australia: Simon & Schuster, 1996.

Davies, Judy. *Planning to Move, Moving to Plan. Living with Developmental Dyspraxia in New Zealand.* Christchurch, New Zealand: Dyspraxia Support Group of N.Z. (Inc.), 1997.

Davis, Ronald D., with Eldon M. Braun. *The Gift of Dyslexia. Why Some of the Brightest People Can't Read and How They Can Learn.* Burlingame, Calif.: Ability Workshop Press, 1994.

Erasmus, Udo. *Fats that Heal, Fats that Kill.* Burnaby, BC, Canada: Alive Books, 1993.

Ewin, Jeannette. *The Fats We Need to Eat. Essential Fatty Acids. Feeling Healthy, Looking Young.* London: Thorsons, 1995.

Feingold, B. F. *Why Your Child Is Hyperactive.* New York: Random House, 1975.

Flick, Grad L., Ph.D. *ADD/ADHD Behavior-Change Resource Kit. Ready-to-Use Strategies & Activities for Helping Children with Attention Deficit Disorder.* West Nyack, N.Y.: The Center for Applied Research in Education, 1998.

Goldish, Meish. *Everything You Need to Know About Dyslexia.* New York: The Rosen Publishing Group, 1998.

Guyer, Barbara P. *The Pretenders. Gifted People Who Have Difficulty Learning.* Homewood, Ill.: High Tide Press, 1997.

Hallowell, Edward M., M.D., and John J. Ratey, M.D. *Driven to Distraction. Recognizing and Coping with Attention Deficit Disorder from Childhood through Adulthood.* New York: Touchstone, 1995.

Henderson, S. E., and D. A. Sugden. *Movement Assessment Battery for Children.* London: The Psychological Corporation, Harcourt Brace and Company, 1992.

Hills, Sandra, N.D., and Pat Wyman, M.A. *What's FOOD Got to Do with It? 101 Natural Remedies for Learning Disabilities.* Windsor, Calif.: The Center for New Discoveries in Learning, 1997.

Ingersoll, Barbara D., Ph.D. *Distant Drums, Different Drummers. A Guide for Young People with ADHD.* Bethesda, Md.: Cape Publications, 1995.

Ingersoll, Barbara D., Ph.D., and Sam Goldstein, Ph.D. *Attention Deficit Disorder and Learning Disabilities. Realities, Myths and Controversial Treatments.* New York: Main Street Books/Doubleday, 1993.

Jacobson, Jane, ed., *The Dyslexia Handbook 1998.* Reading, England: British Dyslexia Association, 1998.

Kaufman, Lorna N., Ph.D., and Pamela Hook, Ph.D. *The Dyslexia Puzzle: Putting the Pieces Together.* Newton, Mass. International Dyslexia Society, New England branch, 1998.

Kelleher, Kelly, J.; Thomas K. McInerny; William P. Gardner; et al. "Increasing identification of psychosocial problems: 1979–1996." *Pediatrics* 105 (2000): 1313–1321.

Kelly, Kate, and Peggy Ramundo. *You Mean I'm Not Lazy, Stupid or Crazy?!* New York: Simon & Schuster, 1993.

Krebs, Dr. Charles, and Jenny Brown. *A Revolutionary Way of Thinking. From a Near-Fatal Accident to a New Science of Healing.* Melbourne, Australia: Hill of Content Publishing Co., 1998.

Levinson, Harold N., M.D. *Dyslexia. A Scientific Watergate. Dyslexia: How and Why Countless Millions Are Deprived of Breakthrough Medical Treatment.* Lake Success, N.Y.: Stonebridge Publishing, 1994.

Ley-Jacobs, Beth M., Ph.D. *DHA: The Magnificent Marine Oil.* Temecula, Calif.: BL Publications, 1999.

Macintyre, Christine. *Dyspraxia in the Early Years.* London: David Fulton Publishers, 2000.

Munden, Alison, and Jon Arcelus. *The AD/HD Handbook.* London: Jessica Kingsley Publishers, 1999.

Nadeau, Kathleen G. *Help4ADD@HighSchool.* Bethesda, Md.: Advantage Books, 1998.

Nosek, Kathleen. *The Dyslexic Scholar. Helping Your Child Succeed in the School System.* Dallas: Taylor Publishing, 1995.

O'Shea, John, and Jenny Dalton. *Dyslexia: How Do We Learn?* Melbourne, Australia: Hill of Content Publishing Co., 1994.

Portwood, Madeleine. *Developmental Dyspraxia. Identification and Intervention. A Manual for Parents and Professionals.* London: David Fulton Publishers, 1999.

Ramsden, Melvyn. *Putting Pen to Paper.* Crediton, Devon, England: Southgate Publishers, 1992.

———. *Rescuing Spelling.* Crediton, Devon, England: Southgate Publishers, 1993.

Richardson, A. J.; A. M. McDaid; C. M. Calvin; et al. "Reduced behavioural and learning problems in children with specific learning difficulties after supplementation with highly unsaturated fatty acids: a randomised, double blind, placebo-controlled trial." Federation of Neuroscience Societies (FENS). Brighton, UK meeting FENS 2000, June 24–28, 2000.

Reichenberg-Ullman, Judyth, N.D., M.S.W., and Robert Ullman, N.D. *Ritalin-Free Kids. Safe and Effective Homeopathic Medicine for ADD and other Behavioral and Learning Problems.* Rocklin, Calif.: Prima Publishing, 1996.

Rief, Sandra, M.A. *The ADD/ADHD Checklist. An Easy Reference for Parents & Teachers.* Paramus, N.J.: Prentice Hall, 1997.

Rose, Colin, and Malcolm J. Nicholl. *Accelerated Learning for the 21st Century.* New York: Dell, 1998.

Salter, Robin, and Ian Smythe, eds. *The International Book of Dyslexia.* London: World Dyslexia Network Foundation and European Dyslexia Association, 1997.

Schmidt, Michael A. *Smart Fats. How Dietary Fats and Oils Affect Mental, Physical and Emotional Intelligence.* Berkeley, Calif.: Frog, Ltd., 1997.

Simopoulos, Artemis P., M.D., and Jo Robinson. *The Omega Diet.* New York: HarperPerennial, 1999.

Smith, Dr. Joan M. *You Don't Have to Be Dyslexic.* Sacramento, Calif.: Learning Time Books, 1996.

Sudderth, David B., M.D., and Joseph Kandel, M.D. *Adult ADD: The Complete Handbook.* Rocklin, Calif.: Prima Publishing, 1997.

Temple, Robin. *Your Child: Dyslexia. Practical and Easy-to-Follow Advice.* Boston: Element Books, 1998.

Umansky, Warren, Ph.D., and Barbara Steinberg Smalley. *ADD: Helping Your Child. Untying the Knot of Attention Deficit Disorders.* New York: Warner Books, 1994.

Vail, Priscilla L. *About Dyslexia. Unraveling the Myth.* Rosemont, N. J.: Modern Learning Press, 1990.

Vitale, Barbera Meister. *Unicorns Are Real. A Right-Brained Approach to Learning.* Torrance, Calif.: Jalmar Press, 1982.

Wallace, Ian. *You & Your ADD Child. Practical Strategies for Coping with Everyday Problems.* Sydney, NSW, Australia: Harper-Collins, 1996.

Weingartner, Paul L. *ADHD Handbook for Families. A Guide to Communicating with Professionals.* Washington, D.C.: Child & Family Press, 1999.

West, Thomas G. *In the Mind's Eye. Visual Thinkers, Gifted People with Learning Difficulties, Computer Images, and the Ironies of Creativity.* New York: Prometheus Books, 1991.

Wodrich, David L., Ph.D. *Attention Deficit Hyperactivity Disorder. What Every Parent Wants to Know.* Baltimore, Md.: Paul H. Brookes Publishing, 1994.

Zimmerman, Marcia, C.N. *The A.D.D. Nutrition Solution. A Drug-Free 30-Day Plan.* New York: Henry Holt & Company, 1999.


## ARTICLES AND SCIENTIFIC PAPERS

Aeschbach, R.; J. Loliger; B. C. Scott, et al. "Antioxidant actions of thymol, carvacrol, 6-gingerol, gingerone and hydroxytyrosol." *Food Chemical Toxicology* 32 (1994): 31–36.

Agostoni, Carlo, et al. "Docosahexaenoic acid status and development quotient of healthy term infants." *Lancet* 346 (September 2, 1995): 638.

Al, M.D.M.; A.C. van Houwelingen; and G. Hornstra. "The effect of pregnancy on the cervonic acid (docosahexaenoic acid) status of mothers and their newborns." Second International Congress of International Society for Study of Fatty Acids and Lipids. Washington, D.C., June 8–11, 1995.

———. Long-chain polyunsaturated fatty acids, pregnancy, and pregnancy outcome. *American Journal of Clinical Nutrition* 71 (2000): 285S–291S.

Anderson, J. W.; B. M. Johnstone; and D. T. Remley. "Breast-feeding and cognitive development: a meta-analysis." *American Journal of Clinical Nutrition* 70 (1999): 525–535.

Andraca, I., and R. Uauy. "Breast feeding for optimal mental development." *World Review of Nutrition and Dietetics* 78 (1995): 1–27.

Appel, L. J.; E. R. Miller; A. J. Seidler; and P. K. Whelton. "Does supplementation of diet with fish oil reduce blood pressure? Meta-analysis of controlled clinical trials." *Archives of Internal Medicine* 153 (1993): 429–438.

Ayres, A. J. "Sensory integration and learning disorders." Los Angeles: Western Psychological Services, 1972.

————. "Sensory Integration and Praxis Tests." Los Angeles: Western Psychological Services, 1979.

Baker, S. M. "A biochemical approach to the problem of dyslexia." *Journal of Learning Disabilities* 18 (1985): 581–584.

Bang, H. O., and J. Dyerberg. "Plasma lipids and lipoproteins in Greenlandic west coast Eskimos." *Acta Medica Scandinavica* 192 (1972): 85–94.

————. "Lipid metabolism, atherogenesis, and haemostasis in Eskimos: the role of the prostaglandin-3 family." *Haemostasis* 8 (1979): 227–233.

Barkley, R. A. "Predicting the response of Hyperkinetic Children to Stimulant Drugs: A Review." *Journal of Abnormal Child Psychology* 4 (1976): 327–348.

Barkley, R. A., and J. V. Murphy. "Treating Attention-Deficit Hyperactivity Disorder: Medication and Behavior Management Training." *Pediatric Annals* 20 (1991): 256–266.

Benton, David. "Fatty Acid Intake and Cognition in Healthy Volunteers." Presented at the NIH Workshop on Omega-3 Essential Fatty Acids and Psychiatric Disorders, 1998.

Biederman, J.; S. V. Faraone; E. Mick; et al. "Clinical correlates of ADHD in females: findings from a large group of girls ascertained from pediatric and psychiatric referral sources."

*Journal of the American Academy of Child and Adolescent Psychiatry* 38 (1999): 966–975.

Birch, D. G.; E. E. Birch; D. R. Hoffman; and R. D. Uauy. "Retinal development in very-low-birth-weight infants fed diets differing in omega-3 fatty acids." *Investigative Ophthalmology and Visual Science* 33 (1992): 2365–2376.

Birch, E. E.; D. G. Birch; D. R. Hoffman; and R. Uauy. "Dietary essential fatty acid supply and visual acuity development." *Investigative Ophthalmology and Visual Science* 33 (1992): 3242–3253.

Birch, Eileen E.; Sharon Garfield; Dennis R. Hoffman; et al. "A randomized controlled trial of early dietary supply of long-chain polyunsaturated fatty acids and mental development in term infants." *Developmental Medicine & Child Neurology* 42 (2000): 174–181.

Birch, Eileen E.; Dennis R. Hoffman; Ricardo Uauy; et al. "Visual acuity and the essentiality of docosahexaenoic acid and arachidonic acid in the diet of term infants." *Pediatric Research* 44 (1998): 201–209.

Boehm, G.; M. Borte; H. J. Bohles; et al. "Docosahexaenoic and arachidonic acid content of serum and red blood cell membrane phospholipids of preterm infants fed breast milk, standard formula supplemented with n-3 and n-6 long-chain polyunsaturated fatty acids." *European Journal of Pediatrics* 155, no. 5 (1996): 410–416.

Brenner, R. R. "Nutritional and hormonal factors influencing desaturation of essential fatty acids." *Progress in Lipid Research* 20 (1981): 41–47.

Broadhurst, C. Leigh; Stephen C. Cunnane; and Michael A. Crawford. "Rift Valley lake fish and shellfish provided brain-specific nutrition for early homo." *British Journal of Nutrition* 79 (1998) 3–21.

Burgess, J. R. "Attention Deficit Hyperactivity Disorder, observational and interventional studies." NIH Workshop on Omega-3 Essential Fatty Acids and Psychiatric Disorders; National Institutes of Health, Bethesda, Md., September 2–3, 1998.

Burgess, J. R.; L. Stevens; W. Zhang; and L. Peck. "Long-chain polyunsaturated fatty acids in children with attention-deficit hyperactivity disorder." *American Journal of Clinical Nutrition* 71 (2000): 327S–330S.

Burr, M. L.; A. M. Fehily; J. F. Gilbert; et al. "Effects of changes in fat, fish and fibre intakes on death and myocardial reinfarction: diet and reinfarction trial (DART)." *Lancet* 2 (1989): 757–761.

Carlson, S. E.; S. H. Werkman; P. G. Rhodes; and E. A. Tolley. "Visual-acuity development in healthy preterm infants: effect of marine oil supplementation." *American Journal of Clinical Nutrition* 58 (1993): 35–42.

Chapkin, R. S. "Reappraisal of the Essential Fatty Acids." In *Fatty Acids in Foods and Their Health Implications,* ed. C. K. Chow. New York: Marcel Dekker, Inc.: 1992.

Christiansen, O, and E. Christiansen. "Fat consumption and schizophrenia." *Acta Psychiatrica Scandinavica* 78 (1988): 587–591.

Chu, Sidney. *Dyspraxia* (conference report, edited notes). *Dyslexia Review.* 1995.

Colquhoun, I., and S. Bunday. "A lack of essential fatty acids as a possible cause of hyperactivity in children." *Medical Hypotheses* 7 (1981): 673–679.

Conners, C. K. "Dyslexia and the Neurophysiology of Attention." In *Perspectives on Dyslexia,* vol. 1., ed. GTh Pavlidis. Chichester, England: John Wiley & Sons, 1990, pp. 163–195.

Corkum, P.; R. Tannock; and H. Moldofsky. "Sleep disturbances in children with attention-deficit/hyperactivity disorder." *Journal of the American Academy of Child and Adolescent Psychiatry* 37 (1998): 637–646.

Coyle, Joseph T. "Psychotropic drug use in very young children." Editorial. *Journal of the American Medical Association* 283 (2000): 1059–1060.

Crawford, M. A. "The role of essential fatty acids in neural development: implications for perinatal nutrition." *American Journal of Clinical Nutrition* 57 (1993): 703S–710S.

Crawford, M. A.; K. Costeloe; W. Doyle; et al. "Essential Fatty Acids in Early Development." In *Polyunsaturated Fatty Acids in Human Nutrition,* eds. U. Bracco and R. J. Deckelman. New York: Raven Press, 1992, pp. 93–110.

Crawford, M. A.; W. Doyle; A. Leaf; et al. "Nutrition and neurodevelopmental disorders." *Nutrition and Health* 9 (1993): 81–97.

Cunnane, S. C.; L. S. Harbige; and M. A. Crawford. "The importance of energy and nutrient supply in human brain evolution." *Nutrition and Health* 9 (1993): 219–235.

D'Alonzo, Bruno. "Identification and education of students with attention deficit hyperactivity disorder." *Preventing School Failure* 40 (1996): 88.

DeFries, J. C., et al. "Colorado Reading Project: An Update." In *The Reading Brain: The Biological Basis of Dyslexia,* eds. D. Duane and D. Gray. Parkton, Md.: York Press, 1991.

DeFries, J. C., and Maricela Alarcon. "Genetics of specific reading disability." *Mental Retardation and Developmental Disabilities Research Reviews* 2 (1996): 39–47.

De Logneril, M.; S. Renaud; N. Mamelle; et al. "Mediterranean alpha-linolenic acid-rich diet in secondary prevention of coronary heart disease." *Lancet* 143 (1994): 1454–1459.

"Diagnosis and Treatment of Attention Deficit Hyperactivity Disorder." NIH Consensus Statement Online 1998 November 16–18; 16(2): 1–37.

Dykman, R. A., and P. T. Ackerman. "Attention deficit disorder and specific reading disability: separate but often overlapping disorders." *Journal of Learning Disabilities* 24 (1991): 96–103.

Eden, G. F.; J. W. VanMeter; J. M. Rumsey; et al. "Abnormal processing of visual motion in dyslexia revealed by functional brain imaging." *Nature* 382 (1996): 66–69.

Edwards, Rhian W., and Malcolm Peet. "Essential Fatty Acid Intake in Relation to Depression." In *Phospholipid Spectrum Disorder in Psychiatry,* eds. M. Peet, Iain Glen, and David F. Horrobin. Carnforth, England: Marius Press, 1999.

Elia J.; P. J. Ambrosini; and J. L. Rapoport. "Treatment of attention-deficit-hyperactivity disorder among children in public schools." *American Journal of Public Health* 89 (1999): 1359–1364.

Eyestone, L. L., and R. J. Howell. "An Epidemiological Study of Attention Deficit Hyperactivity Disorder." In *Psychopharmacology: The Fourth Generation of Progress,* eds. F. Bloom and D. Kupfer. New York: Raven Press, 1994, pp. 1643–1652.

Fagerheim, T.; P. Raeymaekers; F. E. Tonnessen; et al. "A new gene (DYX3) for dyslexia is located on chromosome 2." *Journal of Medical Genetics* 36 (9) (1999): 664–669.

Feingold, B. F. "Hyperkinesis and learning disabilities linked to the investigation of artificial food colors and flavors." *Journal of Learning Disabilities* 9 (1976): 19–27.

Fleisler, S. J., and R. E. Anderson. "Chemistry and metabolism of lipids in the vertebrate retina." *Progress in Lipid Research* 22 (1983): 79–131.

Fletcher, J. M.; B. R. Foorman; S. E. Shaywitz; and B. A. Shaywitz. "Conceptual and Methodological Issues in Dyslexia Research: A Lesson for Developmental Disorders." In *Neurodevelopmental Disorders: Contributions to a New Framework from the Cognitive Neurosciences,* ed. H. Tager-Flusberg. Cambridge, Mass: MIT Press (in press).

Flynn, J. M., and M. H. Rahbar. "Prevalence of reading failure in boys compared with girls." *Psychology in the Schools* 31 (1994): 66–71.

Friedman, Susan. "Dad Learns to Read: How Russell Cosby Overcame Dyslexia." *Family Education Network* (1998). Internet: www.familyeducation.com

Galaburda, A., and M. Livingstone. "Evidence for a magnocellular defect in developmental dyslexia." *Annals of the New York Academy of Sciences* 682 (1993): 71–81.

Grosser, G. S., and C. S. Spafford. "Light sensitivity in peripheral retinal fields of dyslexic and proficient readers." *Perceptual Motor Skills* 71 (1990): 467–477.

Goldstein, Sam. "Attention-deficit/hyperactivity disorder: implications for the criminal justice system." *FBI Law Enforcement Bulletin* 66, no. 6 (1997): 11.

Hamazaki, Tomohito, et al. "The effect of docosahexaenoic acid on aggression in young adults." *Journal of Clinical Investigation* 97, no. 4 (1996): 1129–1134.

Haslum, M. N. "Predictors of dyslexia?" *Irish Journal of Psychology* 10 (1989): 622–630.

Hawkes, Ellen. "I had to grow up fast." *Parade Magazine,* January 8, 1989.

Heird, W. C.; T. C. Prager; and R. E. Anderson. "Docosahexaenoic acid and the development and function of the infant retina." *Current Opinions in Lipidology* 8 (1997): 12–16.

Hibbeln, J. R. "Fish consumption and major depression." *Lancet* 351 (1998): 1213.

———. "Long-chain Polyunsaturated Fatty Acids in Depression and Related Conditions." In *Phospholipid Spectrum Disorder in Psychiatry,* eds. M. Peet, Iain Glen, and David F. Horrobin. Carnforth, England: Marius Press, 1999.

Hibbeln, J. R., and N. Salem. "Dietary polyunsaturated fatty acids and depression: when cholesterol does not satisfy." *American Journal of Clinical Nutrition* 62 (1995): 1–9.

———. "Cholesterol lowering drugs alter polyunsaturated fatty acid levels." *Biological Psychiatry* 40 (1996): 686–687.

Hinshelwood, James. "Word-blindness and visual memory." *Lancet* 2 (1895): 1564–1570.

Hoagwood, K.; K. J. Kelleher; M. Feil; and D. M. Comer. "Treatment services for children with ADHD: a national perspective." *Journal of the American Academy of Child and Adolescent Psychiatry* 39 (2000): 198–206.

Holdcroft, A.; A. Oatridge; V. J. Hajnal; and G. M. Bydder. "Changes in brain size in normal pregnancy." *Journal of Physiology* 498 (1997): 54P.

Holland, B.; A. A. Welch; I. D. Unwin; et al. *McCance and Widdowson's The Composition of Foods.* Cambridge, England: Royal Society of Chemistry and Ministry of Agriculture Fisheries and Food, 1991.

Holman, R. T. "The slow discovery of the importance of w3 essential fatty acids in human health." *Journal of Nutrition* 128 (1998): 427S–433S.

Holman, R. T.; S. B. Johnson; and P. L. Ogburn. "Deficiency of essential fatty acids and membrane fluidity during pregnancy and lactation." *Proceedings of the National Academy of Science* 88 (1991): 54835–54839.

Horrobin, David F. "A Speculative Overview: The Relationship between Phospholipid Spectrum Disorders and Human Evolution." In *Phospholipid Spectrum Disorder in Psychiatry*, eds. M. Peet, Iain Glen, and David F. Horrobin. Carnforth, England: Marius Press, 1999.

———. "The Phospholipid Concept of Psychiatric Disorders and Its Relationship to the Neurodevelopmental Concept of Schizophrenia. In *Phospholipid Spectrum Disorder in Psychiatry*, eds. M. Peet, Iain Glen, and David F. Horrobin. Carnforth, England: Marius Press. 1999.

Horrobin, D. F., and C. N. Bennett. "New gene targets related to schizophrenia and other psychiatric disorders: enzymes, binding proteins and transport proteins involved in phospholipid and fatty acid metabolism." *Prostaglandins, Leukotrienes and Essential Fatty Acids* 60(3) (1999): 141–167.

Horrobin, D. F.; A. I. M. Glen; and C. J. Hudson. "Possible relevance of phospholipid abnormalities and genetic interactions in psychiatric disorders: the relationship between dyslexia and schizophrenia." *Medical Hypotheses* 45 (1995): 605–613.

Horwood, L. John, and David M. Fergusson. "Breast feeding and later cognitive and academic outcomes." *Pediatrics* 101 (1998): 1–7.

Hynd, G. W.; A. R. Lorys, M. Semrud-Clikeman; et al. "Attention-deficit disorder without hyperactivity: a distinct behavioural and neurocognitive syndrome." *Journal of Child Neurology* 6 (suppl) (1991): 35–41.

Innis, S. M. "Essential fatty acids and growth and development." *Progress in Lipid Research* 30 (1998): 39–103.

Jensen, P. S.; L. Kettle; M. T. Roper; et al. "Are stimulants overprescribed? Treatment of ADHD in four U.S. communities." *Journal of the American Academy of Child and Adolescent Psychiatry* 38 (7) (1999): 797–804.

Jensen, Peter S., M.D., and Jennifer D. Payne. "Behavioral and Medication Treatments for Attention Deficit Hyperactivity Disorder: Comparisons and Combinations." Paper presented to NIH Consensus Conference, November 1998.

Jones, J.; M. Barrett; B. Byers; et al. "Prisoners of Time: Report of the National Education Commission on Time and Learning." Washington, D.C.: National Education Commission on Time and Learning, 1994.

Kadesjo, B., and C. Gillberg. "Attention deficits and clumsiness in Swedish 7-year-old children." *Developmental Medicine and Child Neurology* 40 (1998): 796–804.

———. "Developmental coordination disorder in Swedish 7-year-old children." *Journal of the American Academy of Child and Adolescent Psychiatry* 38 (1999): 820–828.

Kang, J. X., and A. Leaf. "The cardiac antiarrhythmic effects of polyunsaturated fatty acids." *Lipids* 31 (1996): S41–S44.

Kozielec, T., and B. Starobrat-Hermelin. "Assessment of magnesium levels in children with attention deficit hyperactivity disorder (ADHD)." *Magnesium Research* 10 (2) (1997): 143–148.

Kromhout, D.; E. B. Bosschieter; and C de L. Coulander. "The inverse relation between fish consumption and 20-year mortality from coronary heart disease." *New England Journal of Medicine* 312 (1985): 1205–1209.

LeFever, G. B.; K. V. Dawson; and A. Morrow. "The extent of drug therapy for attention deficit-hyperactivity disorder among children in public schools." *American Journal of Public Health* 89 (1999): 1359–1364.

Livingstone, M. S.; G. D. Rosen; F. W. Drisland; and A. M. Galaburda. "Physiological and anatomical evidence for a magnocellular deficit in developmental dyslexia." *Proceedings of the National Academy of Sciences* 88 (1991): 7943–7947.

Lucas, A.; R. Morley; T. J. Cole; et al. "Breast milk and subsequent intelligence quotient in children born pre-term." *Lancet* 339 (1992): 261–264.

Lyon, G. R. "Toward a definition of dyslexia." *Annals of Dyslexia* 45 (1995): 3–27.

Lyon, G. R., and L. C. Moats. "Critical conceptual and methodological considerations in reading intervention research." *Journal of Learning Disabilities* 30 (1997): 578–588.

MacDonell, L. E. F.; F. K. Skinner; M. E. Macdonald; et al. "Neuropsychological, visual and essential fatty acid assessments of adults with dyslexic type problems." Poster presented to dyslexia conference in Athens 1997.

Makrides, M.; M. Neumann; K. Simmer; et al. "Are long-chain polyunsaturated fatty acids essential nutrients in infancy?" *Lancet* 345 (1995): 1463–1468.

Mannuzza, S., and R. G. Klein. "Predictors of outcome of children with attention-deficit hyperactivity disorder." *Child and Adolescent Psychiatric Clinics of North America* 1 (1992): 567–578.

Ministry of Agriculture, Fisheries and Food. *Fatty Acids Supplement to McCance and Widdowson's The Composition of Foods.* Cambridge and London: Royal Society of Chemistry and Ministry of Agriculture Fisheries and Food, 1998.

Missiuna, C., and H. Polatajko. "Developmental dyspraxia by any other name: are they all just clumsy children?" *American Journal of Occupational Therapy* 49, no. 7 (1995): 619–627.

Mitchell, E. A.; M. G. Aman; S. H. Turbott; and M. Manku. "Clinical characteristics and serum essential fatty acid levels in hyperactive children." *Clinical Pediatrics* 26 (1987): 406–411.

Moffit, T. E. "Juvenile delinquency and attention deficit disorder: boys' development trajectories from age 3 to age 15." *Child Development* 61 (1990): 893–910.

Moffit, T. E., and H. L. Harrington. "Delinquency Across Development: The Natural History of Antisocial Behaviour in the Dunedin Multidisciplinary Health and Development Study." In *The Dunedin Study: From Birth to Adulthood*, eds. W. Stanton, and P. Silva. Oxford, England: Oxford University Press, 1994.

Moffit, T. E., and P. A. Silva. "Self-reported delinquency: neuropsychological deficit and history of attention deficit disorder." *Journal of Abnormal Psychology* 16 (1988): 553–569.

Morgan, W. Pringle "A case of congenital word-blindness." *British Medical Journal*, November 7, 1896, p. 1378.

Morley, Ruth. "Nutrition and cognitive development." *Nutrition* 14 (1998): 752–754.

"National Institutes of Health Consensus Development Conference Statement; diagnosis and treatment of attention-deficit/hyperactivity disorder." *Journal of the American Academy of Child and Adolescent Psychiatry* 39 (2000): 182–193.

Offord, D. R., and K. J. Bennett. "Conduct disorder: long-term outcomes and intervention effectiveness." *Journal of the American Academy of Child and Adolescent Psychiatry* 33 (1994): 1069–1077.

Oski, Frank A. "What we eat may determine who we can be." *Nutrition* 13 (1997): 220–221.

Pennington, B. F., and J. W. Gilger. "How Is Dyslexia Transmitted?" In *Developmental Dyslexia: Neural, Cognitive and Genetic Mechanisms*, eds. C. H. Chase, G. D. Rosen, and G. F. Sherman. Baltimore, Md.: York Press, 1996, pp. 41–62.

Polatajko, Helene; A. M. Fox; and Cheryl Missiuna. "An international consensus on children with developmental coordination disorder." *Canadian Journal of Occupational Therapy* 62, no. 1 (1995)

Richardson, A. J.; A. M. McDaid; T. Easton; et al. "Is There a Deficiency of Long-Chain Polyunsaturated Fatty Acids in Dyslexia?" NIH Workshop on Omega-3 Essential Fatty Acids in Psychiatric Disorder; National Institutes of Health, Bethesda, Md., September 2–3, 1998.

Richardson, Alexandra J.; I. Jane Cox; Janet Sargentoni; and Basant K. Puri. "Abnormal cerebral phospholipid metabolism in dyslexia indicated by phosphorus-31 magnetic resonance spectroscopy." *NMR in Biomedicine* 10 (1997): 309–314.

Richardson, Alexandra J.; Terese Easton; Anna C. Corrie; et al. "Is developmental dyslexia a fatty acid deficiency syndrome?"

Accepted for publication in the *Proceedings of the Nutrition Society*, 58 (1) (1999).

Richardson, Alexandra J.; Terese Easton; Ann Marie McDaid; et al. "Essential Fatty Acids in Dyslexia: Theory, Evidence and Clinical Trials." In *Phospholipid Spectrum Disorder in Psychiatry*, eds. M. Peet, Iain Glen, and David F. Horrobin. Carnforth, England: Marius Press, 1999.

Richardson, Alexandra J., and Basant K. Puri. "Brain Phospholipid Metabolism in Dyslexia Assessed by Magnetic Resonance Spectroscopy." In *Phospholipid Spectrum Disorder in Psychiatry*, eds. M. Peet, Iain Glen, and David F. Horrobin. Carnforth, England: Marius Press, 1999.

Roush, W. "Arguing over why Johnny can't read." *Science* 267 (1995): 1896–1898.

Sanders, T.A.B., and S. Reddy. "The influence of a vegetarian diet on the fatty acid composition of breast milk and the essential fatty acid status of the infant." *Journal of Pediatrics* 120 (1992): S71–S77.

Satterfield, J.; J. Swanson; A. Schel; et al. "Prediction of antisocial behavior in attention-deficit disorder boys from aggression/defiance scores." *Journal of the American Academy of Child and Adolescent Psychiatry* 33 (1994): 185–190.

Scarborough, H. S. "Early Identification of Children at Risk for Reading Disabilities: Phonological Awareness and Some Other Promising Predictors." In *Specific Reading Disability*, eds. B. Shapiro, P. Accardo, A. Capute. Baltimore, Md.: York Press (in press).

Shaywitz, Sally E. "Dyslexia (current concepts)." *New England Journal of Medicine* 338, no. 5 (1998): 307–312.

Shaywitz, S. E.; J. M. Fletcher; and B. A. Shaywitz. "Issues in the definition and classification of attention deficit disorder." *Topics in Language Disorders* 14 (1994): 1–25.

Shaywitz, Sally E.; Bennett A. Shaywitz; et al. "Functional disruption in the organization of the brain for reading in dyslexia." *Proceedings of the National Academy of Sciences* 95 (1998): 2636–2641.

Shaywitz, S. E.; B. A. Shaywitz; J. M. Fletcher; and M. D. Escobar. "Prevalence of reading disability in boys and girls: results of the Connecticut Longitudinal Study." *Journal of the American Medical Association* 264 (1990): 998–1002.

Simopoulos, A. P. "Omega-3 Fatty Acids Part II: Epidemiological Aspects of Omega-3 Fatty Acids in Disease States." In *Handbook of Lipids in Human Nutrition*, eds. A. Sinclair and R. Gibson. Boca Raton, Fla.: CRC Press, 1996, pp. 318–324.

Starobrat-Hermelin, B., and T. Kozielec. "The effects of magnesium physiological supplementation on hyperactivity in children with attention deficit hyperactivity disorder (ADHD). Positive response to magnesium oral loading test." *Magnesium Research* 10 (2) (1997): 149–156.

Stein, J., and V. Walsh. "To see but not to read: the magnocellular theory of dyslexia." *Trends in Neuroscience* 20 (1997): 147–152.

Stevens, Laura J., and John R. Burgess. "Essential Fatty Acids in Children with Attention-Deficit/Hyperactivity Disorder." In *Phospholipid Spectrum Disorder in Psychiatry*, eds. M. Peet, Iain Glen, and David F. Horrobin. Carnforth, England: Marius Press, 1999.

Stevens, L. J.; Sydney S. Zentall; Marcey L. Abate; et al. "Omega-3 fatty acids in boys with behavior, learning, and health problems." *Physiology & Behavior* 59 (1996): 915–920.

Stevens, L. J.; S. S. Zentall; J. L. Deck; et al. "Essential fatty acid metabolism in boys with attention-deficit hyperactivity disorder." *American Journal of Clinical Nutrition* 62 (4) (1995): 761–768.

Stordy, B. Jacqueline. "Benefit of docosahexaenoic acid supplements to dark adaptation in dyslexics." *Lancet* 346 (1995): 385.

———. "Dyslexia, attention deficit disorder, dyspraxia—do fatty acids help?" *Dyslexia Review* 9 (1997): 5–7.

———. "Dark adaptation, motor skills, docosahexaenoic acid and dyslexia." *American Journal of Clinical Nutrition* 71 (2000): 323S–326S.

———. "The Fats of Life." Paper presented at the 30th International Convention of the Australian Institute of Food Science and Technology, Perth, Western Australia, May 4–8, 1997.

———. "Long-chain Fatty Acids in the Management of Dyslexia and Dyspraxia." In *Phospholipid Spectrum Disorder in Psychiatry*, eds. M. Peet, Iain Glen, and David F. Horrobin. Carnforth, England: Marius Press, 1999.

Styler, Trudie. "Growing Pains (Parents and Dyspraxic Children)." *Harper's Bazaar*, December 1, 1994, p. 69.

Swanson, J. M., et al., "Effect of stimulant medication on children with attention deficit disorder: a review of reviews." *Exceptional Children* 60 (1993): 154–162.

The MTA Cooperative Group. "A 14-month randomized clinical trial of treatment strategies for attention-deficit/hyperactivity disorder." *Archives of General Psychiatry* 56 (1999): 1073–1086.

Uauy, R.; P. Peirano; D. Hoffman; et al. "Role of essential fatty acids in the function of the developing nervous system." *Lipids* 31 (1996): S167–S176.

Vargha-Khadem, F.; K. E. Watkins; C. J. Price; et al. "Neural basis of an inherited speech and language disorder." *Proceedings of the National Academy of Sciences* 95, no. 21 (1998): 12695–12700.

Venuta, A.; C. Spano; L. Laudizi; et al. "Essential fatty acids: The effect of dietary supplementation among children with recurrent respiratory infections." *Journal of International Medical Research* 24, no. 4 (1996): 325–330.

Viadero, Debra. "Cracking the Code." *Teacher Magazine on the Web*, www.edweek.org, January 1998.

Voigt, Robert G.; Antolin Llorente; Marcia, C. Berretta. "Effect of dietary docosahexaenoic acid (DHA) supplementation does not improve the symptoms of attention-deficit/hyperactivity disorder (AD/HD)," part 2 of 2. *Pediatric Research* 45, no. 4 (1999): 17A.

Wainwright, P. E. "Do essential fatty acids play a role in brain and behavioral development?" *Neuroscience and Behavioral Reviews* 16 (1992): 193–205.

Willats, P.; J. S. Forsyth; M. K. DiModugno; et al. "Effect of long-chain polyunsaturated fatty acids in infant formula on problem solving at 10 months of age." *Lancet* 352 (1998): 688–691.

———. "Influence of long-chain polyunsaturated fatty acids on infant cognitive function." *Lipids* 33, no. 10 (1998): 973–979.

Willett, Walter C., et al. "Intake of *trans* fatty acids and risk of coronary heart disease among women." *Lancet* 341 (1993): 581–585.

Wolff, P. H.; G. F. Michel; M. Ovrut; and C. Drake. "Rate and timing precision of motor coordination in developmental dyslexia." *Developmental Psychology* 26 (1990): 349–359.

Woodbury, M. M., and M. A. Woodbury. "Neuropsychiatric development: two case reports about the use of dietary fish oils and/or choline supplementation in children." *Journal of the American College of Nutrition* 12, no. 3 (1993): 239–245.

Zametkin, A. J., et al. "Cerebral glucose metabolism in adults with hyperactivity of childhood onset." *New England Journal of Medicine* 323 (1990): 1361–1366.

Zametkin, A. J.; W. Liotta; C. J. Vaidya; et al. "Selective effects of methylphenidate in attention deficit hyperactivity disorder: a functional magnetic resonance study." *Proceedings of the National Academy of Sciences* 95 (1998): 14494–14499.

Zametkin, A. J.; and J. L. Rapoport. "Neurobiology of attention deficit disorder with hyperactivity: where have we come in 50 years?" *Journal of the American Academy of Adolescent Psychiatry* 26 (1987): 676–686.

Zito, Julie Magno; Daniel J. Safer; Susan dosReis; et al. "Trends in the prescribing of psychotropic medications to preschoolers." *Journal of the American Medical Association* 283 (2000): 1025–1030.

## TV

Vargas, Elizabeth, and Forrest Sawyer. "Bill Cosby's Dyslexia Crusade." *ABC Good Morning America,* July 7, 1997.

# LIST OF REFERENCES
# SPECIFICALLY FOR
# MEDICAL PROFESSIONALS

Burgess, J. R.; L. Stevens; W. Zhang; and L. Peck. "Long-chain polyunsaturated fatty acids in children with attention-deficit hyperactivity disorder." *American Journal of Clinical Nutrition* 71 (2000): 327S–330S.

Colquhoun, I., and S. Bunday. "A lack of essential fatty acids as a possible cause of hyperactivity in children." *Medical Hypotheses* 7 (1981): 673–679.

Richardson, Alexandra J.; I. Jane Cox; Janet Sargentoni; and Basant K. Puri. "Abnormal cerebral phospholipid metabolism in dyslexia indicated by phosphorus-31 magnetic resonance spectroscopy." *NMR in Biomedicine* 10 (1997): 309–314.

Richardson, Alexandra J.; Terese Easton; Anna C. Corrie; et al. "Is developmental dyslexia a fatty acid deficiency syndrome?" *Proceedings of the Nutrition Society,* 1998.

Richardson, Alexandra J.; Terese Easton; Ann Marie McDaid; et al. "Essential Fatty Acids in Dyslexia: Theory, Evidence and Clinical Trials." In *Phospholipid Spectrum Disorder in Psychiatry*, eds. M. Peet, Iain Glen, and David F. Horrobin. Carnforth, England: Marius Press, 1999.

Richardson, Alexandra J., and Basant K. Puri. "Brain Phospho-
   lipid Metabolism in Dyslexia Assessed by Magnetic Reso-
   nance Spectroscopy." In *Phospholipid Spectrum Disorder in
   Psychiatry*, eds. M. Peet, Iain Glen, and David F. Horrobin.
   Carnforth, England: Marius Press, 1999.
Stevens, Laura J., and John R. Burgess. "Essential Fatty Acids in
   Children with Attention-Deficit/Hyperactivity Disorder." In
   *Phospholipid Spectrum Disorder in Psychiatry*, eds. M. Peet,
   Iain Glen, and David F. Horrobin. Carnforth, England:
   Marius Press, 1999.
Stevens, L. J.; Sydney S. Zentall; Marcey L. Abate; et al. "Omega-3
   fatty acids in boys with behavior, learning, and health prob-
   lems." *Physiology & Behavior* 59 (1996): 915–920.
Stevens, L. J.; S. S. Zentall, J. L. Deck; et al. "Essential fatty acid
   metabolism in boys with attention-deficit hyperactivity disorder." *American Journal of Clinical Nutrition* 62, no. 4 (1995):
   761–768.
Stordy, B. Jacqueline. "Benefit of docosahexaenoic acid supplements to dark adaptation in dyslexics." *Lancet* 346 (1995): 385.
———. "Dyslexia, attention deficit disorder, dyspraxia—do fatty
   acids help?" *Dyslexia Review* 9 (1997): 5–7.
———. "Dark adaptation, motor skills, docosahexaenoic acid
   and dyslexia." *American Journal of Clinical Nutrition* 71
   (2000): 323S–326S.
———. "Long-chain Fatty Acids in the Management of Dyslexia
   and Dyspraxia." In *Phospholipid Spectrum Disorder in Psychiatry*, eds. M. Peet, Iain Glen, and David F. Horrobin. Carnforth, England: Marius Press, 1999.
Voigt, Robert G.; Antolin Llorente; Marcia C. Berretta; et al.
   "Effect of dietary docosahexaenoic acid (DHA) supplementation does not improve the symptoms of attention-deficit/
   hyperactivity disorder (AD/HD), part 2 of 2. *Pediatric Research* 45, no. 4 (1999): 17A.

# INDEX

An "f" or "t" following a page number indicates that information is found in a figure or table.

## ABOUT THE AUTHORS

B. JACQUELINE STORDY, PH.D., is an internationally recognized figure in the field of nutrition. She has served on advisory committees established by the British government and the European Community. For many years, she was senior lecturer of nutrition in the School of Biological Sciences at the University of Surrey. She was also director of nutrition degrees at the University of Surrey, managing Europe's largest undergraduate nutrition program. She is an affiliate member of the British Dietetic Association and a member of the Nutrition Society. She lives with her family in Guildford, England.

MALCOLM J. NICHOLL is a journalist who has written extensively on nutrition and education. His previous books include *The Amazing Micro Diet*, *The Loser-Friendly Diet*, and *The Network Strategy*. His most recent book *Accelerated Learning for the 21st Century* was coauthored with Colin Rose. He lives in San Diego, California.